The Tao of Immortality

The Four Healing Arts and the Nine Levels of Alchemy

Mantak Chia
and William U. Wei

T0333536

Destiny Books
Rochester, Vermont • Toronto, Canada

Destiny Books
One Park Street
Rochester, Vermont 05767
www.DestinyBooks.com

Destiny Books is a division of Inner Traditions International

Originally published in Thailand in 2016 by Universal Tao Publications under the title *Cosmology of Taoist Immortality: Universal Healing Tao System*

Library of Congress Cataloging-in-Publication Data

Names: Chia, Mantak, 1944– author.
Title: The Tao of immortality : the four healing arts and the nine levels of alchemy / Mantak Chia and William U. Wei.
Other titles: Cosmology of Taoist immortality
Description: Rochester, Vermont : Destiny Books, 2018. | Originally published under title: Cosmology of Taoist immortality : universal healing Tao system. Thailand : Universal Tao Publications, 2016. | Includes bibliographical references and index.
Identifiers: LCCN 2017013506 (print) | LCCN 2017052295 (e-book) | ISBN 9781620556702 (pbk.) | ISBN 9781620556535 (e-book)
Subjects: LCSH: Taoism. | Healing—Religious aspects—Taoism. | Alchemy—Miscellanea.
Classification: LCC BL1920 .C2577 2018 (print) | LCC BL1920 (e-book) | DDC 299.5/1444—dc23
LC record available at https://lccn.loc.gov/2017013506

Printed and bound in the United States by Versa Press, Inc.

10 9 8 7 6 5 4 3 2 1

Text design and layout by Priscilla Baker
This book was typeset in Garamond Premier Pro with Futura, Present, and Sho used as display typefaces

Photographs by Sopitnapa Promnon

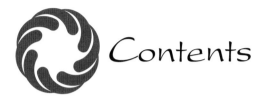

Contents

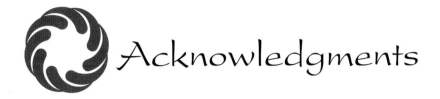

Acknowledgments

The Universal Healing Tao Publications staff involved in the preparation and production of *The Tao of Immortality: The Four Healing Arts and the Nine Levels of Alchemy* extend our gratitude to the many generations of Taoist masters who have passed on their special lineage, in the form of an unbroken oral transmission, over thousands of years. We thank Taoist Master Yi Eng (White Cloud) for his openness in transmitting the formulas of Taoist Inner Alchemy.

We offer our eternal gratitude to our parents and teachers for their many gifts to us. Remembering them brings joy and satisfaction to our continued efforts in presenting the Universal Healing Tao system. For their gifts, we offer our eternal gratitude and love. As always, their contribution has been crucial in presenting the concepts and techniques of the Universal Healing Tao.

We wish to thank the thousands of unknown men and women of the Chinese healing arts who developed many of the methods and ideas presented in this book. We offer our gratitude to Bob Zuraw for sharing his kindness, healing techniques, and Taoist understandings.

We thank the many contributors essential to this book's final form: The editorial and production staff at Inner Traditions/Destiny Books for their efforts to clarify the text and produce a handsome new edition of the book and Nancy Yeilding for her line edit of the new edition.

Thanks to Juan Li for the use of his beautiful and visionary paintings, illustrating Taoist esoteric practices. We wish to thank Colin Drown,

Otto Thamboon, our senior instructors Felix Senn and Andrew Jan, and Charles Morris for their editorial work on the earlier edition of this book. For their efforts on the first edition of this book, we thank our Thai production team: Hirunyathorn Punsan, Sopitnapa Promnon, Udon Jandee, and Suthisa Chaisam.

Putting the Universal Healing Tao System into Practice

The practices described in this book have been used successfully for thousands of years by Taoists trained by personal instruction. Readers should not undertake the practice without receiving personal transmission and training from a certified instructor of the Universal Healing Tao, since certain of these practices, if done improperly, may cause injury or result in health problems. This book is intended to supplement individual training by the Universal Healing Tao and to serve as a reference guide for these practices. Anyone who undertakes these practices on the basis of this book alone, does so entirely at his or her own risk.

The meditations, practices, and techniques described herein are not intended to be used as an alternative or substitute for professional medical treatment and care. If any readers are suffering from illnesses based on mental or emotional disorders, an appropriate professional health care practitioner or therapist should be consulted. Such problems should be corrected before you start training.

Neither the Universal Healing Tao nor its staff and instructors can be responsible for the consequences of any practice or misuse of the information contained in this book. If the reader undertakes any exercise without strictly following the instructions, notes, and warnings, the responsibility must lie solely with the reader.

This book does not attempt to give any medical diagnosis, treatment, prescription, or remedial recommendation in relation to any human disease, ailment, suffering, or physical condition whatsoever.

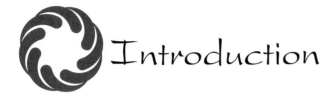# Introduction

After over sixty years of study, practice, and research of the Immortal Tao and Living Tao of the Universal Healing Tao practices, Master Chia is excited to share his insights, discoveries, and observations with his devoted students, instructors, and Taoist practitioners in this book. The long journey of discovering the Tao that Master Chia has taken, starting from his chance meeting as a teenager with his initial Taoist master, Yi Eng (White Cloud), through his young adulthood, marriage, fatherhood, and retiring years, has revealed interesting, informative, and intriguing nuances and subtleties of the Taoist practices. They have evolved into the Universal Healing Tao system, a living organism with its roots in the information and formulas coming from millennia of Taoist masters, reintroduced by Mantak Chia through his world tours to North America, Western and Eastern Europe, Asia, Africa, and Australia and his teaching for over fifty years.

The Universal Healing Tao system will continue to evolve through his thousands of Taoist students and the hundreds of Taoist masters and instructors he has trained. At age seventy-three Master Chia is continuing to tour and has set up a global internet broadcasting station at Tao Garden, his Chiang Mai Universal Healing Tao training facility and health resort, to do live broadcasting around the world on the Tao and its mystical Way. In addition, he will continue to share new formulas to explain and practice the Tao through courses, books, booklets, audios, DVDs, and Chi Cards corresponding to the books, as well as online with his websites: www.universal-healing-tao.com, www.tao-garden.com, and www.mantak-chia.com. Numerous future books will expand the Living Tao, Chi Nei Tsang, Cosmic Healing, and Immortal Tao practices. The Universal Healing Tao system will carry on for millennia to come, to share the understandings and practices of the Tao in over thirty different languages for global understanding.

In the realms of time, human beings have been influenced by mystical schools, religions, governments, and now corporations. They have convinced us to give them our time and energy (essence) for the good of others, but mostly for themselves. They promise they will take care of us or save us. When we give everything to them, we have no time or energy left for ourselves, and in the end we have nothing except their promises. Other systems taught us how to cultivate and grow our energy like a seed into a tree, but after a while they told us they needed our energy for the good of others, and they convinced us to give them our tree for their own use. And other systems even went further, showing us how to grow flowers from our tree, and after the flowers blossomed, they told us to pick them for their beauty and sell them to others.

But the Tao teaches us not only how to plant (root) and grow our seed (energy or essence) into a tree, but also how to sexually cultivate the seed so that it can flower and bear fruit, without losing our essence (original seed). Our tree (cultivated energy) will bear abundant fruit, which we can share with others who are sincere and deserving. Now think: in each piece of fruit that we bear, how many seeds are in it to share? So if we cultivate our original seed in the Tao, instead of giving it away as other systems advise, we are able to share thousands of seeds for the good of others, and never lose our original seed (essence). This is the Way of the Tao that is explained and taught in the Universal Healing Tao system.

To know the Tao is to feel the Tao, and the only way to feel the Tao is to practice the Tao. So the hardest part of the Tao is finding someone who is practicing the Tao and is willing to teach you the Taoist practices so you can feel the Tao. Master Chia has dedicated this book to giving his thousands of students and fellow Taoist practitioners the fine points,

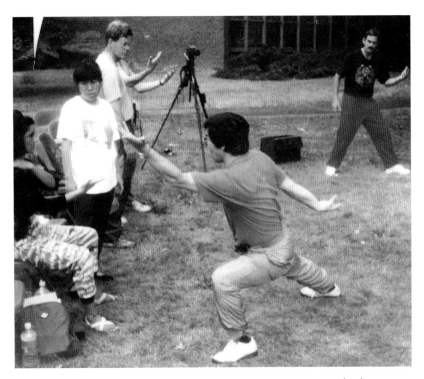

Master Chia teaching Tai Chi Chi Kung to W. U. Wei and others at
Summer Retreat in Big Indian, New York, July 1986

emphasis, and correct focus of the Universal Healing Tao practices for
their enjoyment and self-discovery. This book gives you a unique perspective and understanding of Master Chia's practices and techniques
and helps you to find the key meaning of the Universal Healing Tao
practices in a simplified way. The book reveals the concept, theory, and
purpose of the Tao. It also makes clear why you should practice, how
you should practice, and when and where you should practice. From it
you will learn where the energy and intention of the Tao originates and
where it is going, how you connect with the Tao, and your purpose for
being on the earth plane from a Taoist perspective.

We come into this world with nothing and we leave this world with
nothing. No riches, monuments, accomplishments, wealth, or relationships go with us. So why should we waste all our time and energy trying

to accumulate these things? In physical death our spirit and soul bodies leave the physical body because they can no longer function in a body that has deteriorated through physical and emotional abuse, accidents, degenerative diseases, or simply old age. What we take with us is our consciousness (spirit and soul). So does it not make sense that we should devote time every day to develop and cultivate our consciousness, which is the only thing that we take with us at physical death? This is the message of the Tao explained in this book by Master Chia.

It is important to know that this book is an accelerated course in the ancient Taoist teachings. In ancient times, the knowledge that is shared in this book took years to grasp. Reading and studying the book will give you a lot of information, but it is only that, information. It is not yet wisdom. A portion of wisdom means experience and only time can give you what you need in that regard.

Once you have the concept of the Tao, it will create your desire to do your daily Taoist practice. And that is the only way you will get the results you are looking for. Our mental (concept) body controls our emotional (desire) body, and our emotional (desire) body controls our physical (manifestation) body. As Napoleon Hill stated in his book *Think and Grow Rich,* what the mind can conceive and believe, the mind can achieve. Once you have developed your daily Taoist practice, another law of the universe is activated: spaced repetition for lasting transformation. For example, if you dump a bucket of water on a rock, you will get a big splash but nothing will happen to the rock, except it will be cleaner. But if you take that same bucket of water and tilt it just enough so one drop at a time hits the rock (spaced repetition), before all the water is out of the bucket it will split the rock. Similarly, the water is your internal energy or effort and the rock is what you want to accomplish with your daily Taoist practice. Through your daily Taoist practice you will gradually achieve self-awareness and ultimately enlightenment. With this self-awareness you will be able to make conscious decisions for your daily life and discover who you really are and where you are going.

After you have established a daily morning Taoist practice of five to ten minutes, then you can start to integrate these practices in your daily life effortlessly. This is why Master Chia has developed simplified forms of the Universal Healing Tao practices, revealed in this book—so that you can utilize them in your daily life at work, in your community, and in your family or personal life. This all starts with slowing down your mind, or your "monkey mind" as the Taoists refer to it, because it gets you into a lot of mischief, or doing unnecessary action. Slowing down the mind helps you to make conscious choices. This simplifies your life: instead of reacting to life situations, you have time to consciously choose action that is beneficial to you and others.

Master Chia shares his wisdom and understandings of the Universal Healing Tao practices so you can integrate them into your daily life to be a better person for yourself and others. Master Chia gives you this unique concept and purpose of the Tao, which gives purpose and meaning to your life's journey. Once you practice the Tao you receive balance and harmony from the universe as you align yourself to its flow and oneness. You become a better human being because your attitude, purpose, and intention change for the betterment of yourself and others. As you become better in balance and harmony within your own circumstances, the energy you generate internally from these Taoist practices will unintentionally and indirectly be shared with others, going beyond your circumstances of race, creed, citizenship, childhood, and DNA.

The Universal Healing Tao system can be broken down into Four Healing Arts, which encompass the original Nine Levels of Inner Alchemy. The Four Healing Arts are as follows:

- Living Tao practices for transformation of your emotional body
- Chi Nei Tsang Practices for transformation of your physical body
- Cosmic Healing practices for transformation of your energy body
- Immortal Tao practices for transformation of your spiritual body

In this book Master Chia further explains each of these Four Healing Arts with their more than 240 formulas and outlines a short, simplified version of key practices to integrate into your daily life.

This book begins with a presentation of the fundamentals of Taoist Immortality as well as Inner Alchemy, changing one substance into another energetically, which is the whole basis of the Universal Healing Tao system. Then Master Chia gives you the evolution of the Universal Healing Tao system from the core of the original Nine Levels of Taoist Inner Alchemy taught to him by his first Taoist master, Yi Eng, over sixty years ago.

The Nine Levels of Taoist Inner Alchemy are as follows:

1. Primordial Force Activation
2. Sexual Alchemy
3. Fusion Alchemy
4. Lesser Enlightenment of Kan and Li
5. Greater Enlightenment of Kan and Li
6. Greatest Enlightenment of Kan and Li
7. Sealing of the Five Senses
8. Congress of Heaven and Earth
9. Reunion of Heaven and Man

Each level is explained in great detail in concept, theory, and purpose with its Inner Alchemy formulas, including basic, intermediate, and advanced formulas.

With great delight and pleasure, I acknowledge the opportunity Master Chia has given me to assist him in organizing his thoughts and discoveries of the simplified Taoist concepts and practices revealed in this book. I have been his student, friend, collaborator, and a dedicated practitioner of the Universal Healing Tao system over the last thirty years. So it gives me great joy to collaborate with him again on this major book leading to Taoist Immortality. It has been a grand journey of personal self-discovery with the Universal Healing Tao practices and discovery of the Tao and its mystical Way with the guidance and tute-lage of Master Mantak Chia. I trust you will enjoy this book with its insights, concepts, and directions into the Universal Healing Tao system as you discover your true self and its destiny.

WILLIAM U. WEI (WEI TZU)
THE PROFESSOR—MASTER OF NOTHINGNESS
THE MYTH THAT TAKES THE MYSTERY OUT OF MYSTICISM

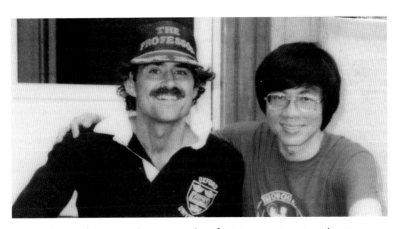

The professor and Master Chia first met at Master Chia's Beginners' Healing Tao Workshop in Toronto, Canada, November 19, 1984.

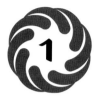

Taoist Fundamentals

The Tao is the natural flow of the universe. It is what makes everything move. The Tao is the life force in everything that we touch, see, smell, hear, and taste. It is the way the river flows, the sun glows, the wind blows, the tree grows, and the way a seed becomes a rose. The Tao is in the air we breathe. It is the very breath that gives us life and the life force within us. You cannot describe or define it; you can only experience and feel it. It is the Primordial Force, Supreme Creator, God, or the Wu Chi, Ultimate Stillness.

The Tao is the power of now. You can be joyful and happy right now. You do not need to wait until you go to heaven; you can find balance in life now. You can do it with practice, appreciation, gratitude, and compassion. You can learn how to delete the pain and suffering by connecting to the Primordial Force. You can learn how to not get sick, through balance, detachment, and understanding. The Tao, the source of all things, is eternal and continually changing. It is the path of direct and divine experience of unconditional love, harmony, and balance, which is its essence. The Tao is the one force that governs the whole universe. The Tao is not a religion, but it embraces all religions. Universal love of the Tao is a direct connection to the Tao in our hearts, our Original Spirit, a spark of our divinity. No other spiritual system is as clear or comprehensive in its use and enhancement of chi, the activating energy of all movement in the universe, the life force of all created things.

Through the Big Bang the physical universe was created with the interaction of yang (supercluster) and yin (dark matter) as it went into a quantum leap, resulting in thousands and thousands of physical things. Primordial Force—an aspect of dark matter, as it is known in modern science—fills the whole universe. Each galaxy contains part of the Primordial Force, especially our galaxy, our solar system, and our planet Earth. Taoist practice evokes the Primordial Force—Former Heaven Essence—in order to reunite it with spirit and soul—Later Heaven Essence—in our body. Everyone has a spirit and soul that contain energy. You receive the spirit and soul from the Primordial Being or Creator. Every day newborn intelligent spirits and souls are created. Because they are like infants, we call them infant spirits and souls. They age, grow, and become part of the universe.

In our galaxy there are 300 billion stars (see fig. 1.1). Clearly something or somebody controls them. This is all the more true when you consider the fact that there are millions or even billions of galaxies. The

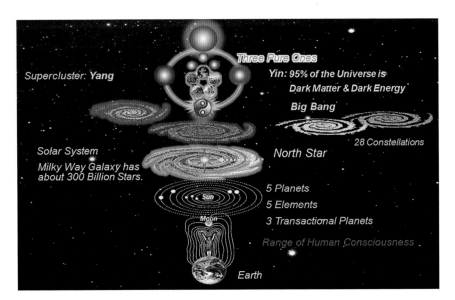

Fig. 1.1. Human observation of the universe

Taoist wants to be part of the universe, so this is of great significance. Every connection in the universe has intelligence; this is precisely what controls the universe. Dark matter and dark energy are about 95 percent of the universe, and the other 5 percent is our physical universe. Our brain cells work within a network of dark matter like the universe. Our spirit and soul have the intelligent energy of the septillion stars in the universe. In fact, they are this intelligent energy, but they need to be trained and educated about who and what they are and where they are going.

OUR LIGHT BODY:
SPIRIT BODY AND SOUL BODY

From the Taoist perspective our light body—which consists of our spirit and soul bodies—enters our physical body. Our spirit is our divinity (free will) and our soul is our identity (persona). Our spirit is the life force that keeps us alive and our soul is our memory body. Our human quality is our spirit body; it is not in our DNA (soul body). We are light bodies (cosmic dust particles, stars of the light); we are divine and inhabit our physical bodies to gain human experiences to develop and cultivate our spirit and soul bodies. All light bodies are equal in their own divinity.

The spirit is our consciousness that connects to the whole (Wu Chi). The soul is our memory, which we carry on from sojourn to sojourn as a part of our light body. The Taoist says we have two deaths—when we physically die and when the last person who knew us physically dies—but our light bodies never die, because energy cannot be destroyed. We were never born and we will never die, because we are divine without beginning or end. That is our consciousness, which gives our physical body life and without which our physical body cannot live. When our physical body breaks down through chronic abuse, degenerative diseases, emotional stress, or age, then our light body can no longer inhabit our physical body and it leaves (ascends); this is physical death, not spiritual death.

Our light bodies collectively created our known universe with a collective thought projected into the emptiness (Wu Chi) and it reflected back, forming our evolving universe (the Big Bang). We were so good at doing this that we forgot who we really are (the forgotten gods). This creative process is reinforced every time we enter the human form because the DNA is so strong that it shocks our memory body and we do not remember anything until we discover, develop, and cultivate our spirit and soul bodies.

Again from a Taoist perceptive, our whole purpose on the earth plane as human beings is to discover our own divinity, which we experience every time we create something from thought (concept), desire (motivation), and manifestation (completion). We literally reenact the original creation process of the universe every time we create something. Look around your room; the same process created everything you see, from clothing, furniture, television, computers, and phone to the building holding them all. Creation requires free will and the ability to think, which separates us from all other living forms on Earth and gives us our divinity, whether we are conscious of it or not. This is not only the ability to think and conceptualize but also the desire to manifest it based not only on survival but also on inspiration.

We receive violet light energy from the North Star (see fig. 1.2). It is the light of wisdom with the ability to access all knowledge. Universal violet light energy has universal intelligence that is interconnected, as

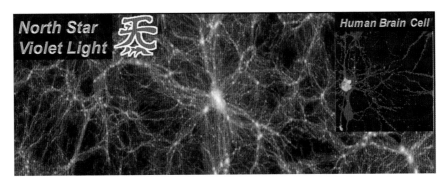

Fig. 1.2. The North Star's violet light and a human brain cell

our brain is connected to our whole body. As above, so below, as the Taoists say, relating the macrocosm and the microcosm. Violet light has the highest healing force that can be programmed. It can be developed to help us to be connected to this vast universe.

Everything is related and connected, but communication is of paramount importance. Every spirit and soul requires violet light for intercommunication. This is important because, for example, in the case of cancer cells, the cells are broken and unable to communicate. Receiving violet light facilitates communication, which leads to better health.

The intelligence of violet light is in the newly born spirit and soul in the human form. The spirit and soul are related to quantum theory. The wave character, the "other half" of the DNA system, was discovered in 1975. It is complementary to the material aspect. This implies that there is a universal system of communication between the cells of the body, a complex system of vibrations ranging in frequency between ultrasound and ultraviolet light. Ultraviolet frequency biosignals "ride" on the spirals of DNA and activate specific codons, the biological information units in the 64-triplet code of DNA. The DNA codons are analogous to the 64 trigram combinations of the I Ching. Falsification of these signals means cancer; their extinction "puts out the light" of the whole body.

We are all connected and there is intelligence in this interconnection. It is shown in the Higgs field theory that establishes the existence of the Higgs boson, which is also known as the "God particle" (see fig. 1.3).

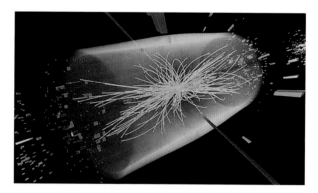

Fig. 1.3. The Higgs field is a fundamental field of crucial importance.

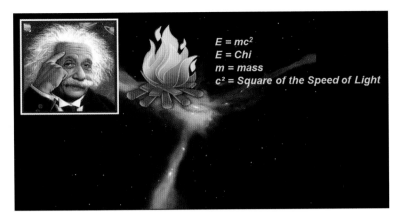

$E = mc^2$
$E = Chi$
$m = mass$
$c^2 = Square\ of\ the\ Speed\ of\ Light$

Fig. 1.4. Albert Einstein's formula: $E = mc^2$

The connection that you have can be programmed. As you develop in your spiritual awareness by knowing more of the Tao, you become more and more connected to the universe. In this way you actually control part of the universe.

Consider Einstein's theory of energy and his famous formula $E = mc^2$, the law of physics stating that energy can neither be created nor destroyed, only transformed (see fig. 1.4).

Understanding this formula will help you understand everything. The spirit that you have will never die, because it is energy. Energy cannot be destroyed, only transformed, so it is immortal, but it has no form. So the spirit and soul need a container that is mass, or our body, to give them form. They are held in the body by our original force or chi (see fig. 1.5).

Fig. 1.5. You come into this world with no spirit or soul, but the body provides a place for them and allows you to discover your mission.

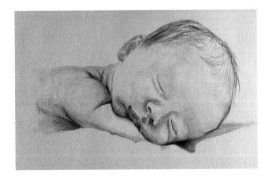

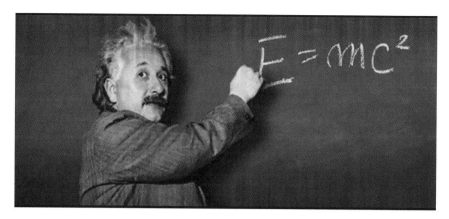

Fig. 1.6. Einstein writing his formula: E = mc²

Albert Einstein's formula tells us the amount of energy a given mass would yield (E = mc²) if it were converted into energy (see fig. 1.6). E = mc²: energy equals mass times the speed of light squared. To find the energy, you multiply the mass by the square of the speed of light (300,000,000 meters per second)—(a very large number); thus, if the mass is 0.111, then 0.111 x 300,000,000 x 300,000,000 = 10,000,000,000,000,000 joules.

FIVE ENLIGHTENMENTS (REALIZATIONS)

According to the Tao, you simply need to understand your original self; the way you were before being pressured to change your true being. What is the original self? First, you have righteousness inside. You have goodness inside you. Of course there are negatives and we must learn to accept them and find a balance. Each of us was born to be consciously connected to the universe and has all the necessary systems to realize our full potential. You have a spirit (conscious body) and a soul (memory body) that enable you to attain your highest form of being and achieve your essence. You are born with a force or power, which constitutes your original programming. All you need to do is know the programming language and techniques to connect to it and you can achieve great joy and happiness. It is that simple.

The language is quite easy to learn because you are born with it. In a way, the programming language is your native tongue. To get in touch with your original being and operating system is actually quite simple. Complicated philosophical systems and endless lectures, talks, and commentaries are not necessary.

What is needed are five realizations:

1. The **first realization** is that you have spirit and soul.
2. The **second realization** is that your spirit is divided into five separate infant spirits within the physical body, which reside energetically in the five vital organs (heart, liver, spleen/stomach, lungs, and kidneys). And each infant spirit corresponds to one of the five elements (fire, wood, earth, metal, and water) (see fig. 1.7 below).
3. The **third realization** is the conscious decision to train and raise your spirit and soul to gain their knowledge and wisdom, taking responsibility for them, knowing that they never die but that if you do not feed (train) them that they will never grow; they will instead remain undeveloped and move on to another physical body after yours dies.
4. The **fourth realization** is that you need to find a practice that will train and grow your spirit and soul; one such practice is our Universal Healing Tao system.
5. The **fifth realization** is that you are born to have a free spirit and soul.

Understanding the First Realization

When we enter human life we are controlled physically by physical force (strength or weapons), mentally by thought control (culture and environment), and spiritually by religions (which condemn you to hell or damnation). Or we can go beyond the karmic wheel, realizing that we have a free spirit and soul that we can train, developing their own understandings and wisdom to enter their place in the divine universe.

The Tao gives us our original operational system at birth. The cosmos or the Creator gives us the blessing of our spirit and soul. The Primordial Force gives us our original life force. The North Star and the earth give us our pulse; we have more than twenty pumps and about fifty-two pulses. The universe is within us, as we live within the universe. The first enlightenment you must achieve is to know you have an infant spirit and soul within you. Know that you have something special deep within your being. You actually feel your spirit and your soul. That is important, just like it would be important to know that you had an infant in your house.

If your spirit and soul energy is depleted and finally runs out, you physically die. So maintaining spirit-soul energy is a matter of life and death. The Bible talks of maintaining oil in the lamp because when the oil is gone the lamp no longer shines. If you are not inclined to believe in the Bible you can just think of your cell phone. If there is no charge or no energy there is no connection.

Understanding the Second Realization

There are five spirits in the body, which are the descendants of the five infant spirits. They are located in the vital organs, each with its own color (see fig. 1.7).

Each of the five spirits is also connected with one of the five elements (see fig. 1.8 on page 18). The descendants of the five infant spirits are the following:

Yuan Shen is our Original Spirit connected with the element fire, located in the heart and small intestine: first in command, with red light (conscious awareness, thought, reason, inspiration, and intuitive insight).

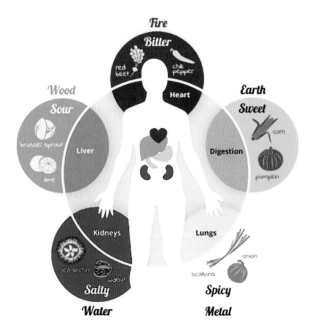

Fig. 1.7. The spirits in our vital organs are different colors.

Hun Shen is our spiritual soul, connected with the element wood and vision, located in the liver and gallbladder: second in command, with green light (dreaming, vision, symbolic imagination, and myth).

Yi Shen is our intention spirit, connected with the element earth and ripening, located in the spleen, stomach, and pancreas: third in command, with yellow light (planning, intention, and action).

Po Shen is connected with the element metal and transformation, located in the lungs and large intestine: fourth in command, with white light (somatic awareness, sensation, organic body processes, and instinctual responses).

Zhi Shen is our willpower, connected with the element water, gestation, birth, and death, located in the kidneys and bladder: fifth in command, with blue light (sexuality and reproduction, magic, obsession and desires, deep sleep, archetypal imagination, fate, collective unconscious, archaic primordial unity, and transformation).

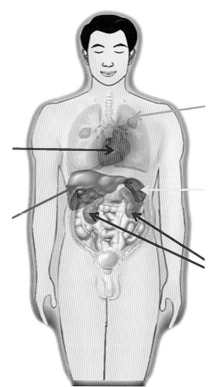

Yuan Shen
Original Spirit
Fire, awareness, reason
Heart, Small Intestine
First in command
Red light

Po Shen
Po soul
Metal, transforming
Lung, Colon
Fourth in command
White light

Yi Shen
Intention spirit
Earth, ripening
Stomach, Pancreas
Third in command
Yellow light

Hun Shen
Hun soul
Wood, vision
Liver, Gallbladder
Second in command
Green light

Zhi Shen
Water, willpower
Kidneys, Bladder
Death, Birth
Fifth in command
Blue light

Fig. 1.8. The spirits and souls of the five vital organs,
descendants of the five infant spirits

Yuan, Hun, and Yi Shen are connected to mind, spirit, and heaven. Po and Zhi are connected to body, matter, and earth. These vital organ spirits have a connection back to the Source.

Understanding the Third Realization

The third realization is to take care of the spirit-soul infants you have within you. It actually consists of a literal decision to take proper care of them. The decision is made regardless of the personal or cosmic expense, in the same manner it is made for taking care of the children you have biologically.

Understanding the Fourth and Fifth Realizations

In ancient times the Taoists talked about the spine being like a building twenty-four stories high. Imagine the connection that would be needed to convey water and electricity from the ground floor to the twenty-fourth floor. The twenty-fourth story is your brain and it similarly needs good connections to the ground. When you awaken in the morning you need to be sure you are grounded. You need to have all of your organs operating and pulsing. You need to be sure that your crown is activated and your antenna operating. Check the basic aspects of your being each morning and you will lead a life that is more alive and more awake. The process is that simple.

You need to remember these principles each day when you awaken: chi is the original force that maintains our life. Always remember that you have an undeveloped spirit and soul. Without development, ignorance will be the result. The spirit and soul have an intrinsic form of intelligence, but it needs to be developed to connect to the universe. That is your goal and the direction you must head. You need a compass and you need to go in the direction of the North Star.

The infant spirit and soul are satisfied by getting candy. The candy is a symbol of food, alcohol, power, drugs, sex, or whatever it is that a lost spirit-soul is seeking. A lost spirit-soul is essentially a hungry ghost. All the hungry ghosts of the universe are like children. This is the worst state you can find yourself in. People who crave power do not want you to grow up and be smarter than them. They want you to remain a child because children are easier to control. Only two things are needed to control a child: candy or a big stick. Do you want candy or do you want the big stick?

Your goal is to become educated, grow up, and recognize your oneness with the universe. In the long run, you want to have wisdom, which cannot be attained in school. Wisdom is only acquired in the stars. That is the fifth attainment. You need a system that will provide enough energy to feed your spirit and soul. The system that you need will provide energy gotten from the earth, the stars, and the heavens. All the planets and stars have inexhaustible energy. The Universal Healing Tao system of Taoist practices with concept, theory, and understandings enables you to transform that energy to your own energy.

Everything is made of particles and each tiny particle contains all the information and memory of the cosmos. In a similar fashion, you can connect to the cosmos and have all the knowledge and wisdom of the cosmos. Energy with no form cannot be enlightened. For enlightenment to be attained a physical form is necessary. That is why humans are in a unique situation, the one that provides an opportunity for enlightenment. Those who do not take advantage of this opportunity will become wandering ghosts or lost souls because they will not have the necessary physical body once they die physically. The impact of this knowledge has significance in many areas and has been established by science.

YIN AND YANG BALANCE

Balance is the key to the Tao; without it the universe would be out of control. The forces that control the universe are yin and yang. If we learn to balance yin and yang we can live in harmony and control our emotional and physical bodies. There are many ways to think of this; for example, the balance needed between emotional intelligence (EQ) and intelligence itself (IQ).

Consider the Tai Chi or yin and yang symbol and what it means (see fig. 1.9). It implies movement, change, and balance. When it moves, yin pushes the yang and yang pushes the yin. This initiates an eternal spinning. Nothing wins and nothing loses. That is the incredible beauty of Tai Chi: nobody wins and nobody loses. There is simply non-stop spinning and balancing, which creates a special harmony. As a result of this the universe is eternal. Without this balance of yin and yang, the universe would cease to be.

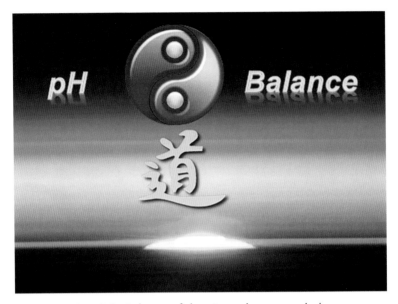

Fig. 1.9. Balance of the yin and yang symbol

This symbol dates back many thousands of years. It was discovered by the Taoists as they realized that the earth spins around itself (see fig. 1.10). There is day and night and everything spins in a circle.

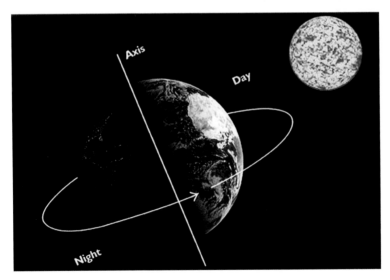

Fig. 1.10. The earth spins around itself.

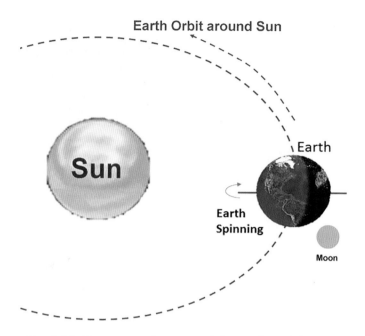

Fig. 1.11. The moon orbits around the earth and the earth orbits around the sun.

Orbiting and spinning are in every part of the universe, from the moon orbiting the earth (28 days), to the earth orbiting the sun (364.5 days), to the sun orbiting around the galaxy (fig. 1.11). Orbits also move in a figure eight, which is a symbol of eternity; it never ends and never begins.

When you focus you can sense the orbits of the sun, moon, and stars; you are aware of their spinning. You can actually feel them inside you and consequently you can feel your internal orbit all the way down to the electron and proton level. The power is within you if you are willing and able to activate it. These orbits are important because, essentially, without orbits there would be no universe. There would be no being, including you. Your internal orbits spin throughout your body along with the universe and keep you connected to it.

You need to learn how to develop your own personal orbit. Once this is accomplished you can then begin to collect energy. The heart is a primary organ in the collection of energy, as is the brain. The main thing to remember is that everything is connected and energy is generated during the process of orbiting through these connections. The connections are not only throughout your entire body; they extend to other people and to the universe.

Taoism is a system of balance, and it is very nature-oriented. We live within nature and try to balance our lives in accord with natural laws of the universe. The balance must start within our own being. A very important aspect to understand is how to utilize energy. When energy moves in orbit, according to Taoist texts, a person is born again. The reason the phrase *born again* is used is because energy is spinning when a fetus is in the mother's womb (see fig. 1.12).

After we are born we have energy, but over time it is lost. As we begin to lose energy, we become more susceptible to sickness. This can be seen even in the physiology of the body: for example, oxygen and carbon dioxide have to find a balance. Negative emotions such as anger or stress cause us to hold on to carbon dioxide, which can lead

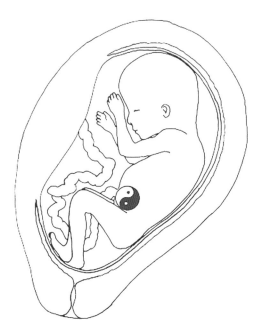

Fig. 1.12. Energy is spinning when a fetus is in the mother's womb.

to sickness. In such situations we need to learn how to relax and let go of the carbon dioxide we are holding; we breathe out and let go of our pain and suffering. One way to look at it is to think of compost. If we put waste products from leftover food or excrement back in the earth, it is life for the earth. Mother Earth uses it for new life and growth. Without this, the earth would be unable to grow anything.

In the same manner we are responsible for Mother Earth, we are responsible for ourselves, including our minds, our emotions, and our behavior. We are responsible for our very being. The best way to handle this and the stress we confront is to release everything back to Mother Earth. Through the practices of the Tao we learn to be self-sufficient and handle situations for ourselves.

THE THREE TAN TIENS

There are three minds or brains in the body, which are known as three tan tiens: one in the brain, one in the heart, and one in the lower abdominal area (see fig. 1.13).

The Chinese have a saying that you should think three times before you act. This saying is based on the ancient wisdom regarding the upper, middle, and lower brains. Often, those that use only the logical brain are narrow-minded because they are only seeing about fifteen degrees of the possible 360 degrees. You need to make sure that the connection between the different brains is clear so that you are more open-minded. The heart is the consciousness and the lower tan tien is the awareness; consciousness and awareness always go together like twins. Information goes through these three brains, which process it, and this is how you learn. Unfortunately most people only use one brain. This is what the Tao and many other ancient teachings try to explain.

To train the spirit and soul we need to understand the way all three minds work as one (see fig. 1.14 on page 26). The awareness mind of the lower tan tien is like a radar that picks up everything in and around

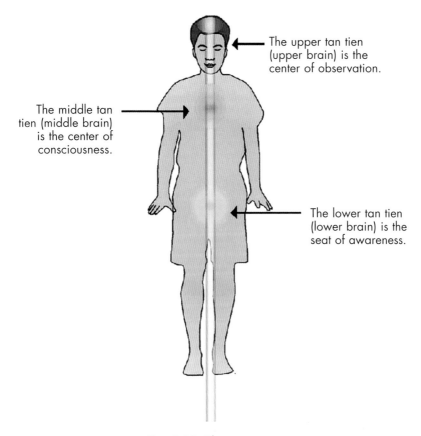

The upper tan tien (upper brain) is the center of observation.

The middle tan tien (middle brain) is the center of consciousness.

The lower tan tien (lower brain) is the seat of awareness.

Fig. 1.13. Three tan tiens

us, which is connected to a monitor so we can view it. It never sleeps. And it is capable of storing all of our excess energy.

The consciousness mind of the middle tan tien or the heart is connected to universal knowledge. It explains to us what the images on the monitor really mean. It also never sleeps. As it is the emotional center, it can lead to confusion if the emotions are not balanced. It gives us feedback. It is not logical or illogical. It is just a reflection.

The observation mind of the upper tan tien or the brain observes the monitor. Its focusing ability of higher mind, eye, and heart offers clarity, but it sleeps when tired, which can be a problem.

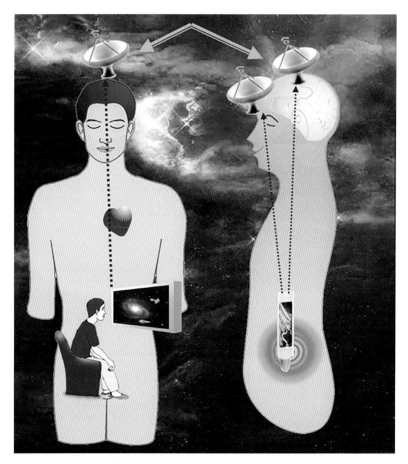

Fig. 1.14. Three minds into one mind: awareness mind,
consciousness mind, and observation mind

Through practice you can bring your three minds into one mind, which will expand your awareness like a radar and let your observing mind watch the monitor in your (lower) tan tien (see fig. 1.15). Then greater awareness, consciousness, and calmness are achieved.

The abdomen is built to store energy. Our intestines serve as a storage battery for our energy in the villi (see fig. 1.16).

The principles of the tan tien are that you begin from the navel and you grow from the navel. A developed tan tien has its own set of senses and is recognized as the sixth sense. You turn three minds into

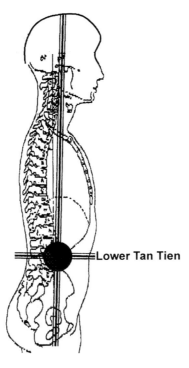

Fig. 1.15. This is the location of the lower tan tien,
often simply referred to as "the tan tien."

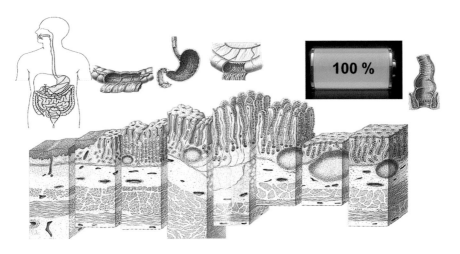

Fig. 1.16. The electrical polarity of our intestines serve as the
storage battery for our energy in the villi.

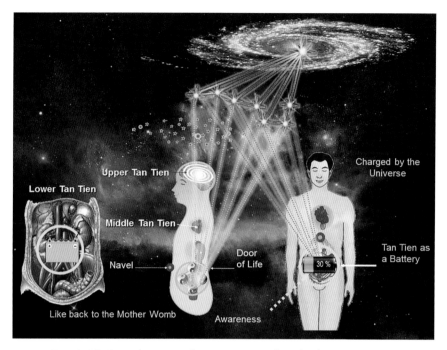

Fig. 1.17. Turn three minds into one mind at the lower tan tien.

one by bringing your energy to the tan tien in the abdominal area (see fig. 1.17).

You were born to be connected to the cosmos and Taoism holds that the connections are easy and important. All you need to understand is that you have an antenna on top of your head. The heart is the key or the on and off switch. You just need to turn your switch on. The only thing that can hold you back from love, joy, and happiness is not turning on the switch, not connecting to the cosmos. The original operating system we are born with facilitates this, but life tends to reprogram us and we lose our original self.

ORIGINAL OPERATING SYSTEM

In order to grasp the foundation of Taoist practice you need to have a deep understanding of the original operating system. For the ancient Taoists, nature was essentially the equivalent to the Tao. This immediately raises the question of what nature is. Nature is something that you are born with and into. This is analogous to a computer and its operating system. After you are born, many things start to try to program you. These influences are, among others, your family, school, religion, and friends.

What must be understood is that there are many belief systems, not just the one that you have been programmed with. We are born to be righteous, free, and connected. Many belief systems have priests and prophets who claim they are the only ones who can talk to God or the Original Source. Many problems result from the claim that there is only one system for the entirety of truth.

The Taoist system trusts that everyone has certain natural truths. One of those truths is that you come into this world with pumps. In fact, you have more than twenty pumps and fifty-two pulses. All this is part of your original operating system. Think of a mountain and water running down the hill. If water only runs downhill and fire only burns upward there are obvious consequences. The result is that one day the water is all gone and the fire has burnt out. However, if you can take the water up above the fire, it can be transformed into steam and the steam goes up. It can then come down in the form of rain and nourish the land, the crops, and everything on Mother Earth. Trees will grow and can be used to rekindle fire.

In the same manner that the mountain is connected to the stream, you are connected to the cosmos. You are born that way. If you are aware of your connection to the cosmos and utilize it, you will be able to nourish your heart, liver, and the other five vital organs. The first step in understanding and applying the natural abilities you are born with is to know and activate your pumping system.

The Energy Waterwheel

The first step that you need to take is to "train the waterwheel" (see fig. 1.18 on page 30). For a detailed explanation of the waterwheel, see

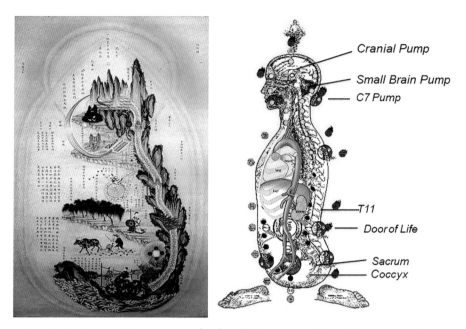

Fig. 1.18. Ancient Taoist waterwheel and the points of the Microcosmic Orbit

the appendix, "The Tang Dynasty Waterwheel Image as an Illustration of the Microcosmic Orbit."

Water has three states: solid, liquid, and steam. When water changes to steam, it goes up. When it condenses, it goes down like rain. The rain is necessary for the growth of trees, plants, and everything living. What this means in your body is that the steam nourishes your brain, cools the heart, and provides growth to the liver, spleen, and stomach. Your land must be plowed in order to grow anything. This simple teaching comes from the ancient Taoists and need not be made complicated or overly esoteric.

Learning how to circulate your energy produces more chi or life force. Essentially this is sexual energy because that is the only type of energy that is capable of transformation. Once you learn this fundamental principle, you are enlightened. Many people practice for years and do not grasp this principle even though it is basic and quite simple. Some people do not have sex and think that they are saintly. Others just think that they are saintly and sex becomes very mysterious. When it becomes mysterious suddenly it also becomes more like a business procedure than enlightenment. The mistake here is that the basic principles of energy are not understood.

Energy, Life, and Death

The Tao, God, or life force gave you a Primordial Force, which is split:

- 25 percent is stored in the sexual organs.
- 25 percent is stored in your kidneys.
- 50 percent remains as your original force, which comes in through the navel at the beginning and remains stationed there (lower tan tien) for the rest of your life.

The original force runs your life and holds your spirit and soul. You do need to eat, breathe, and rest in order to replenish your energy, but it is the original force that powers you. Every time you take a breath or open your eyes you need original force. Each time you think or say something, it is required. The energy in your body is like a bank account or budget. You need to consider how much to spend and what for, as well as to hold some in reserve.

Consequently you should think of your energy as something that you need to budget. Every time you breathe or do anything at all, you use original force; you are tapping into the 50 percent of original force energy. When your light body can no longer function in your physical body because of its deterioration through drugs, accidents, or degenerative diseases, your light body leaves and your physical body dies. That is what death is—not the end of your light body but of your physical body. You must be aware and awake to this fact so that you expend energy wisely.

Kidney energy cannot be transformed into any other type of energy. It is your reserve energy. The force stored in the kidneys is energy for emergencies, for when you are extremely sick. If you have enough stored at the moment of death it will boost your journey to the heavens when you become part of the universe. Unfortunately you can trick your body with substitutes like drugs or alcohol. Many drugs just make your heart and mind race and your respiration increase. This is done at great expense to you. Overdoing drugs or sex or even coffee (worst drug in the West) is not wise. Tricking the kidneys every day with drugs is a recipe for disaster. This actually just kills you slowly because basically you are utilizing your reserve energy.

The Tao teaches that sexual energy is the only kind of energy that can multiply. You can think of it this way: the way the universe operates is that it gives the best energy for creation of a new being. Sex cells contain an astonishing amount of energy. Think of the millions of times the cells split, first to form the fetus and then the ever-changing human being. Over a lifetime, trillions of cells are generated from the single cells contributed by the mother and father. Another way to think of it is that the cells of an individual human being die and replace themselves. Every year you have an entirely new body. Formerly it was believed that this took seven years, but now it is known to take only one year.

It is agreed to by most that two or three children is enough. Most people do not want more than that. This leaves a great deal of untapped sexual energy. A man can have approximately 5,000 ejaculations. Theoretically he could have 5,000 children. A woman has about 400 menstrual cycles. If you do not want children, do not discard your sexual energy but rather transform it. Being able to transform that sexual energy to be utilized for your daily living needs is the key.

Suppose you are very cold and you have a lot of wood. You need to know how to make the wood into fire to warm you. You will have fire only if you know how to start it, which is a formula. By using that formula you will get a fire that will give off the necessary energy. Sexual energy transformation is an easy thing to do. You simply need to remember the well-known formula $E = mc^2$. You have to find the *m*, then you find the *c*.

While this is a very easy proposition, many people do not get it. You cannot just look at your testicles or ovaries and wonder how you are going to transform them. There is always the question of how you transform something that is material into something that is immaterial. In $E = mc^2$ the m is for your sexual organs and the c is for your heart. These are used to create energy. It is that simple. All you need to do is recognize this and develop your Universal Healing Tao energy practices. If you are able to understand the theory and guide yourself through it you will realize that it is real. You will gain the ability to transform the sexual energy for your health and longevity.

As a human being you have the ability to harness your sexual energy. The energy that drives the sexual organs is the fire within you, which you are born with. Energy can only be transformed from one form to another. Science has proven this. A special kind of fire is required to do this. This type of fire is in its essence a sacred fire. You might recall the burning bush in the story of Moses when he is lost in the wilderness for forty years. The bush burned but it was not destroyed. Such a fire is an alchemical fire and it is capable of transformation. In a similar fashion you are capable of being enlightened.

Energy and heat are involved in the Inner Alchemy practices of the Universal Healing Tao (detailed later in this book). Whenever you focus on one part of your body, you should involve the lower tan tien. The heart (middle tan tien) is also an important aspect but it cannot store energy because it will overheat. The brain (upper tan tien) should not overheat either. It is the lower tan tien that stores energy, and when this combines with sexual energy it facilitates bliss. With these practices, it is very important to not think too much, because that cooks the brain and causes serious damage. The same thing can happen to the heart. This reduces the energy in the lower tan tien and brings about serious problems such as chronic fatigue syndrome. Exceptional caution is advised when you are dealing with energy, because it is like electricity.

You can tap into the energy of Mother Earth, which is rejuvenating and replenishing. The key is to push the energy upward, using your organs for assistance. Heat always rises and this is useful to keep in mind. The lower organs are cooler than the higher ones. You can warm the lower organs with the heat from above and also keep the upper organs like the brain and heart cooler by moving the heat downward. As your sexual energy rises, it revitalizes your brain. Your creativity and thinking increase dramatically because you are connected to the universe and are filled with meaningful ideas. To put it another way, to connect to the cosmos you need to utilize your sexual energy to get power.

When you were a child perhaps you played with a magnifying glass. When exposed to the sun, your skin feels warm, but when you use a magnifying glass to condense the energy in one small dot, it is powerful enough to start a fire. This magnification is equivalent to focus, which directs our energy to one specific location. If you focus love, it becomes a loving fire, and your compassion becomes a compassionate fire. This begins with transforming sexual energy utilizing the fire of the tan tien spinning in our midsection.

The sexual energy will then start to transform into the original force, adding life into your life. You are adding more oil into your lamp. The heart is very special because sexual energy can come up to the heart. At that time the sexual energy can be converted into spiritual energy. If you do not comprehend how to transform sexual energy you spend it in a wasteful fashion. It is far better to transform it into spiritual food, which is required for your spirit and soul.

If your spirit and soul bodies are properly nurtured and educated, they grow up to be strong and good as well as self-sufficient. You have the necessary fire and there is no need to wait for it. The various types of energy will gather within you and you can tap into the cosmic forces. These forces are connected to eternity. You do not need to go to church to realize your relationship with the cosmos and its unity. Your spirit and soul are immortal, but they will not grow without the necessary spiritual food.

There is enormous potential within your sexual energy and it has the ability to initiate a positive transformation within you. This is the path toward enlightenment. There is a window of opportunity to transform energy and enlighten the spirit and soul. That opportunity exists when you have a physical body. If your body gets old and dies without being enlightened, the chance at transformation and the creation of additional energy is gone. That is how important the awareness of this practice is. You can compare this to a piece of wood that is exposed to the elements. If nothing is done and it just sits in the sun and rain, it will decay and rot. If it is transformed by lighting it on fire, it creates energy. Similarly, transformed sexual energy can be used to educate and enlighten the spirit and soul, which can become the Immortal One.

According to the concept of sin from the Christian perspective, if you commit a sin God will punish you, perhaps with hell itself. The Taoist view of this matter is different, because there is no such thing as sin. Rather than sin, the Tao talks about balance and imbalance. There is a correlation between enlightenment and physical health. The correlation is this: you need to keep your body fit and healthy, and to do so you need to keep your spirit and soul healthy. Connectedness and balance activate and empower your chi. They assist you in being not only physically healthy and mentally healthy but also spiritually (energetically) healthy.

You need to find a spiritual practice that can supply you enough energy to feed your spirit and soul. If one does not work, simply try another one that you think might be suited to you.

Violet Light

Dark matter cannot be checked or confirmed because there is no polarity. This is equally true of pure yin and pure yang, which are intertwined with dark matter. The ancient Taoists knew of the existence of something that split into yin and yang but they could not prove it. They simply called it the Tao (the space or line between the two extremes). In modern times dark matter and dark energy were

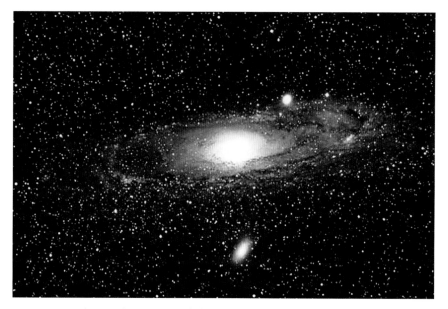

Fig. 1.19. Dark matter and dark energy cover the entire universe,
and this is violet light.

discovered (see fig. 1.19). What the Taoists knew and modern science
has discovered are essentially the same. This is what provides energy to
the cosmos as well as to us as individuals.

According to Taoism, the original force in the heart stores the
Original Spirit. This comes from God, the Supreme Creator, the Tao,
or whatever other terminology you want to use. The point that needs
to be made is that there is a connection with the universe; it is a two-
way connection. The universe connects to us and we connect to the
universe (see fig. 1.20).

The violet light is intelligent energy. The communication between
individual cells uses the violet light. Without violet light there can be no
communication between the cells in your body. If this were to happen
the cells would turn to cancer cells. Your cells require violet light, which
is an integral part of good health. The violet light needs to mix with
loving fire from the heart. The way to get loving fire is to experience
love, joy, and happiness and then condense that fire. With sufficient fire

you can transform internal energy. Everyone has this capability.

It is important to never try to feed your spirit and soul at your body's expense. The key is to utilize your sexual energy, which can be converted without your body paying the price. The energy located in the other organs is finite and capable of being depleted if used unwisely. The procedure for transforming sexual energy is simple. You take the fire that burns within you and put it in your sexual organs. This involves three steps:

1. First you focus, concentrate, and move energy to your lower tan tien.
2. Then you feel love, joy, and happiness, which connect you to the violet light.
3. You will experience the violet light with the activation of sexual energy.

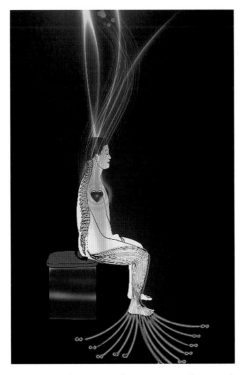

Fig. 1.20. Connecting with yin earth energy and yang heavenly energy

UNDERSTANDING THE WAY
OF THE TAO

To understand the transformational practices covered in this book, you need a basic understanding of Taoist cosmology and the connection of yin and yang, the origin of the five elements and their dynamics. From the Tao arises the complete universe.

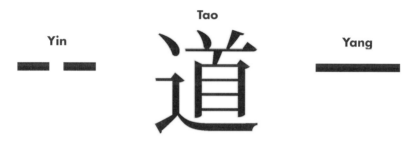

Fig. 1.21. From the Tao arise yin and yang.

When Wu Chi, the Primordial Deep, the Womb of the Mysterious Mother, became pregnant of itself and from its fullness created the one, from the one was created its other, the two, and so yin and yang came into being (see fig. 1.21). And as the two created the three, universal love was introduced between the yin and the yang, which makes one yin and one yang, or one yang and one yin, and even two of the same, yin or yang, stick together.

Wu Chi

Yin 無　　　　　極 Yang

道 生 一 Tao Sheng Yi	Tao gives rise to one.
一生 二 Yi Sheng Er	One gives rise to two.
二生 三 Er Sheng San	Two gives rise to three.
三生萬物 San Sheng Wan Wu	Three gives rise to all things.

At Creation the "Three Pure Ones" arose: the heavenly force, the earth force, and the cosmic force. From the Three Pure Ones issues

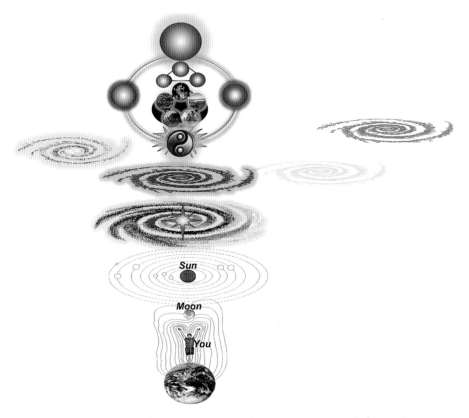

Fig. 1.22. San Sheng Wan Wu: "Three gives rise to all things."

forth the cosmic force, which controls all creation: three yin combine to form Earth, and three yang combine to form Heaven. As Father Heaven and Mother Earth unite, the five elements and eight directions are born. In Taoist tradition it is said that the Three Pure Ones control the five-element star, which shines light of five colors, and in turn controls 400 billion galaxies. According to Taoist cosmology the Three Pure Ones further continue to steer things in Heaven as well as on Earth, ruling the myriad galaxies and our own galaxy, which centers around the polar star. The Three Pure Ones are reflected in our body as the three Elixir Fields or 丹 田 tan tien (tan = elixir; tien = field): the lower, middle, and upper, which correspond to our existence as physical, mental, and spiritual beings.

At the first meeting of Father Heaven and Mother Earth, the Arousing issues from the father, and Completion from the mother. Thus the Arousing (thunder) is the first son, and the Gentle (the wind, wood) is the first daughter. At the second meeting of Father Heaven and Mother Earth, water issues from the father, and fire from the mother. Thus the Abysmal (water) is the middle son, and the Clinging (fire) is the middle daughter. At the third meeting of Father Heaven and Mother Earth, Stillness issues from the father, and Rejoicing from the mother. Thus the Stillness (mountain) is the youngest son, and the Rejoicing (the lake, metal) is the youngest daughter (see fig. 1.23).

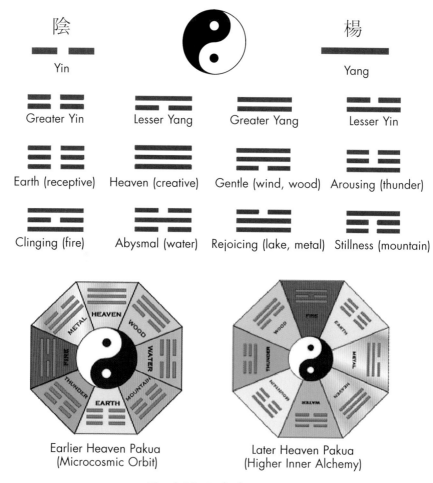

Fig. 1.23. Eight forces

The eight trigrams can be attributed to the eight directions of the pakua in many ways, according to their microcosmic and macrocosmic dynamics. Of these, the Earlier Heaven pakua and the Later Heaven pakua are most important for feng shui and alchemy. The Earlier Heaven pakua, attributed to the legendary Fu Hsi, resembles the eight directions of the globe. The Later Heaven pakua is attributed to King Wen; it reflects the feng shui of the inner body, the organs, and the seasons.

THE FIVE ELEMENTS

In order to learn the Inner Alchemy practices of the Tao, you need to understand the five elements of nature, which have a significant influence on the human body and spirit, as well as the cosmos (see fig. 1.24). These concepts were discovered centuries ago by the

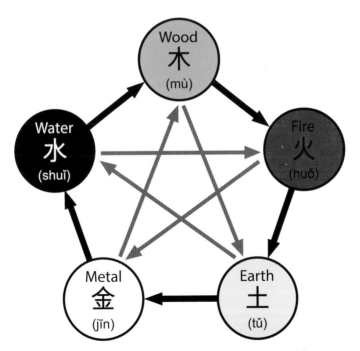

Fig. 1.24. The five elements are part of nature and have a significant influence on the human body and spirit.

Taoist masters. Relative to space they are related to the stars, planets, and cosmic manifestations. These empirically verifiable entities are involved with the five elements: fire, water, wood, metal, and earth. In fact the impact on the universe is the same with you. As you proceed in the practice of the Tao, it is important to keep this in mind. The five elements provide energy to everything. They influence everything including astrology, food, music, medicine, martial arts, and visual arts.

This fundamental basis can be experienced in your own physical body. As you turn inward and recognize the five elements, you feel a link with the universe. Links are profoundly important to everything in life. Simply thinking about links on the internet is a very clear example, but the universal link is also very important in cosmic understanding. As a small universe yourself, you have internal links. You have the five elements within your own body. Externally, you are linked to other people and the universe beyond. It is important to recognize the incredible wisdom that is contained in this structure. One of the beautiful things about this is its simplicity.

First is the fire element, which resides in the heart. The fire element relates to expansion. The season that the fire element links to is summer and its color is red. The emotional portion that relates to the heart is love, joy, and happiness, as well as the negative aspect of hatred, impatience, arrogance, and cruelty. The true Taoist must accept the negative as well as the positive and balance them internally. Internally is where true understanding and wisdom reside.

The Original Spirit resides in the heart. As the spiritual leader, the heart controls the other spirits in your body. All of the spiritual components are linked with every quality of the fire element or heart. They are dressed in red, they look red, and they stay in a red palace. Each of the bodily qualities and the spiritual qualities of the fire element give us a special kind of self-wisdom.

In addition to having internal or personal qualities of the fire element, there are the external aspects of fire, which are the sun, volcanoes, and fire itself. The direction associated with fire is south and it also expands. When you become deeply aware of the fire outside you then it is possible for you to make a connection to this element. One reason for that is due to the fact that fire expands outward to the cosmos. You are linked to fire planets and fire stars.

The fire element burns and becomes the earth element, which is connected to the spleen, pancreas, and stomach. The colors are yellow and brown. It is related to the emotional aspects of worry and anxiety. At the same time, balance and harmony are part of earth's powers. This power is connected to other planets that also have earth powers and balance; you are part of this vision of the cosmos. The earth element has seventy-two days of transitional periods often called Indian summer.

When you dig into the earth, one thing that you will find is metal, and thus earth gives birth to the metal element. The metal element is fall or autumn and has seventy-two days. It is a time for harvesting and collecting. The color of metal is white and is related to the lungs. Some of the emotions associated with metal are courage, sincerity, and righteousness as well as depression, grief, and sadness. Mountains, rain, and lakes contain the power of metal. As the rain comes down the mountain it washes up metals. Metal enriches water.

The water element is connected to the kidneys and the bladder. Its season is winter, which consists of seventy-two days and is a time for retreat and stillness. The color of water is blue. The kidneys store fear and phobias and their related qualities. Willpower is also stored in the kidneys and its spirit is dressed in blue and lives in a blue palace. Realization of this has benefits for this life and leads toward bodily, spiritual, and cosmic health.

Wood is the next element and it is connected with the liver and gallbladder. Its season is spring, and it is green in color. The negative emotions in this element are envy and jealousy. Thinking and planning are a part of the wood element. Spring is a period of seventy-two days and is involved with growth, which makes wood and vitality.

FIVE-ELEMENT RELATIONSHIPS

ELEMENT	ORGANS	EMOTIONS
Wood	Liver, Gallbladder	Anger, Forgiveness
Fire	Heart, Small Intestine	Cruelty, Joy
Earth	Spleen, Stomach	Brooding, Openness
Metal	Lungs, Large Intestine	Sorrow, Courage
Water	Kidneys, Bladder	Fear, Stillness

From a Taoist perspective, this concept relates to one of the most important aspects of the practice, which is balance. In addition the five elements are used to describe relationships between phenomena (see fig. 1.25).

FIVE ELEMENTS

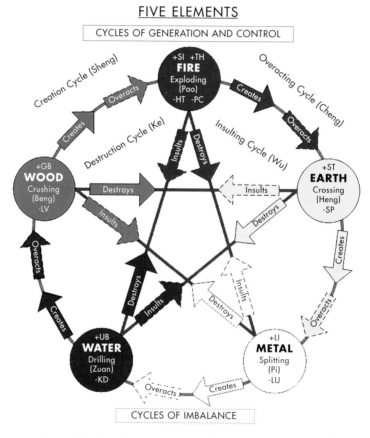

Fig. 1.25. The five elements explain cosmic cycles and relationships among internal organs.

QUALITIES OF THE FIVE ELEMENTS

ELEMENT	COLORS	DIRECTION	ENERGY	SEASON	CLIMATE	YIN/YANG
Fire	Red and Orange	South	Ascending	Summer	Hot	Full Yang
Earth	Yellow and Brown	Center	Stabilizing	Indian summer	Damp	Yin/Yang Balance
Metal	White and Silver	West	Contracting (Internal)	Fall	Cool	Dry New Yin
Water	Black and Blue	North	Descending	Winter	Cold	Full Yin
Wood	Green	East	Expansive (External)	Spring	Warm	Wet New Yang

A true and sincere trust in the five elements leads to wisdom and then enlightenment. Becoming enlightened involves being aware of the interconnectedness of everything. You can look into your own being and find the five elements and ask yourself which ones you see and which one best represents you. You can think of this as knowledge and wisdom. It is esoteric on the one hand but scientific on the other. It is scientific because it actually works if you understand it. You can use this knowledge in your daily life, your emotional life, and your spiritual life, and empirically verify the results. Discovering and comprehending the five elements is a profound and world-changing experience.

ORGAN AND ELEMENT INTERCONNECTIONS

ORGAN	LUNGS	KIDNEYS	LIVER	HEART	SPLEEN	TRIPLE WARMER
Associated Organ	Large intestine	Bladder	Gallbladder	Small intestine	Pancreas Stomach	x
Color	White	Dark blue	Green	Red	Yellow	x
Sound	Sss-s-s-s-s	Choo-oo-oo-oo	Sh-h-h-h-h	Haw-w-w-w-w-w	Who-oo-oo-oo	Hee-e-e-e-e
Positive Emotions	Courage Righteousness	Gentleness Wisdom	Kindness Generosity	Joy Honor Sincerity	Fairness Balance Centering	x
Negative Emotions	Sadness Sorrow Grief	Fear	Anger	Impatience Insincerity	Worry	x
Element	Metal	Water	Wood	Fire	Earth	
Season	Autumn	Winter	Spring	Summer	Indian Summer	x

THE EIGHT IMMORTALS AND SIXTY-FOUR HEXAGRAMS

It is also extremely helpful to know and deeply grasp the Eight Immortals, or eight forces, which correspond to the eight directions. The directions are related to various elements and to organs in the body. The relationship of the Eight Immortals to your own body is very important. The fact is that links and connections might be the most significant part of the Taoist practice.

EIGHT IMMORTALS AND THEIR CONNECTIONS

IMMORTAL	LINKS
Li	Fire, sexuality, and relationships
Kan	Water, especially pure water
Chen	Lightning, thunder, and exercise
Tui	Rain, sleep, and rest
Sun	Wind and emotions
Chien	Heaven and spirituality
Kun	Harmony and digestion
Ken	Mountain and work

The eight forces are representations of nature and the universe. They are used to gather chi into the lower abdomen. Cosmically, they are used to create a more powerful connection with the universe. Each of these forces is represented by a unique trigram combination of three yin and yang lines. Further combinations of the eight primordial forces account for everything in life and the universe.

This is the DNA of the universe and is exactly the same as our own DNA. The sixty-four combinations of the eight primordial forces are the basis of the "world formula," the sixty-four hexagrams of the ancient

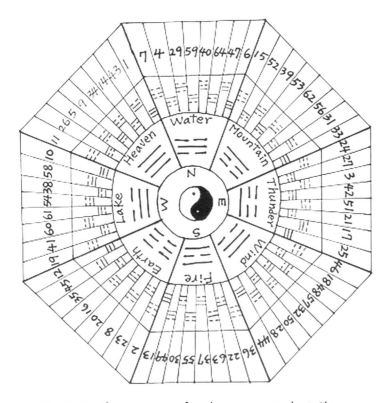

Fig. 1.26. There are sixty-four hexagrams in the I Ching.

Taoist text the I Ching (see fig. 1.26). Their mathematical structure corresponds precisely with the structure of the DNA in all living things, including each one of us humans. This is an amazing correspondence of the insights of the ancient Taoists and the discoveries of modern genetic science.

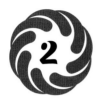

Inner Alchemy Framework

To be a knowledgeable practitioner of the Tao you need to understand the interconnections of the various aspects and particulars of the Tao from the big picture, which needs to be grasped thoroughly. The procedure always starts with making a connection. There are two essential connections. One is to the material world as you know it: the earth, plants, animals, trees, sun, and moon. The second is seemingly more esoteric but is being verified more and more by science. That connection is the effect the North Star has on the earth and consequently the effect it has on you.

We are born with these two connections: one to Heaven (North Star, yang, positive charge) from our crown and the other to Earth (grounding, yin, negative charge) from our tailbone. An analogy to the antenna in your crown might be a cell phone that connects you to people and things like the internet. If you do not have a connection because your battery is dead you have a problem. Some people are born with a type of energy that allows them to make connections. These people are often called prophets because they can talk to God or the cosmos as a result of their special energy or connection. Everyone, through practice, is capable of having a connection to the cosmos.

FEELING THE TAO

To understand the Tao, you must learn to feel the Tao. How you feel the Tao is from above (Heaven) and below (Earth) through your spine (see fig. 2.1).

The Tao teaches us not only balance but the oneness of everything. This unity means that we are connected to every part of our body, to others, to the earth, and heavenly bodies. Everyone was born with this connection. It is as though we have an antenna that connects to the universe, located in the cranium at the spot on the skull where there is an opening at birth. That opening gradually closes as we grow older. The exact spot varies from individual to individual, with some people's pointing more to the back than others. Metaphorically speaking we are born with this connection, which acts like an antenna and all we have to do is turn it on (see fig. 2.2 on page 50).

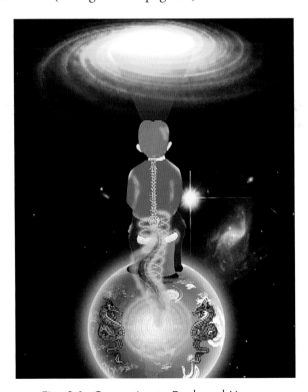

Fig. 2.1. Connection to Earth and Heaven

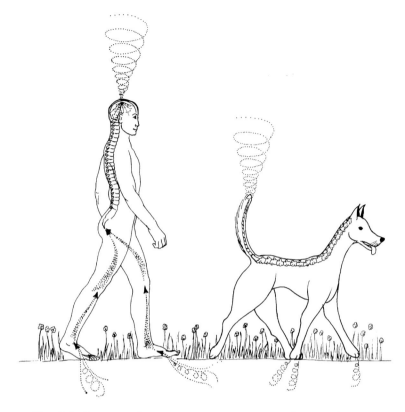

Fig. 2.2. Everyone has an antenna connecting them to the Tao.

Our tailbone and the soles of our feet are the wiring to the earth while our cranium is the heavenly wiring. The earth wiring is negative energy and the heavenly wiring is positive. With the negative and positive connections we get electricity. With this wiring connection of Heaven and Earth we have an internal dragon; when activated, it becomes the Fire Dragon.

Expanded awareness is like having good radar. Radar has a monitor, but it is of no use if there is no one watching it. This is where focus comes in. It is like looking for something on a search engine and getting thousands of results. Without focus and without wisdom, you have no idea about what you are doing. Consciousness is inward while awareness is outward. You need to have both (see fig. 2.3).

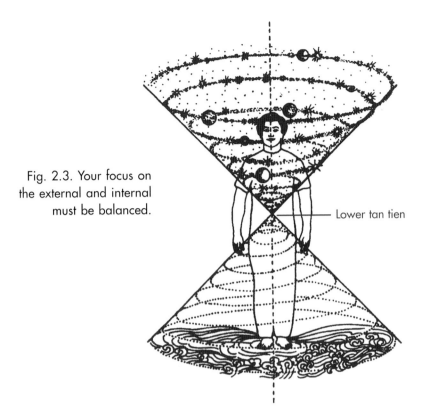

Fig. 2.3. Your focus on the external and internal must be balanced.

Lower tan tien

You live in an inner universe and an outer universe. Wisdom is what makes connecting the two possible. This connection is very important because if you do not have it, then your concentration is split in half. At the same time that you expand your awareness out, you need to be conscious of your inward self. Your awareness can be trained to get better and better. And you can be trained to have many different kinds of consciousness.

The Influences of the North Star

The North Star is critical, not just in terms of the Tao, but in terms of navigation as well. Navigation of the earth as well as understanding where to ground ourselves requires knowing where the North Star is. The influences of the North Star are profound; they include basic aspects such as your pulse and your breathing. Connecting to the North Star is having an awareness of the cosmos that is not just energetic but very practical. You need this connection in order to function and be a happy and balanced person. As you navigate through the stress and problems that modern society brings, you tend to lose a sense of what is important. The North Star lights your path and gives you a direction.

While all the stars and planets are important, the North Star is the most significant star or planet in the cosmos. The earth is being pulled by the North Star, which is substantiated by a lot of evidence. The earth tilts toward the North Star and Southern Cross (see fig. 2.4). It should be noted that the tilt of the earth is changing and this will have a big impact on the temperatures of the poles.

As with the entire teaching of the Tao, everything is connected. There is almost a chain of pulses that originates with the North Star. The North Star affects the earth pulse and the earth pulse affects our pulse (see fig. 2.5). Science has shown that the pulse of the earth affects everything on the earth, including people. In humans there are two separate pulsing systems: the actual pulse and the heartbeat. The puls-

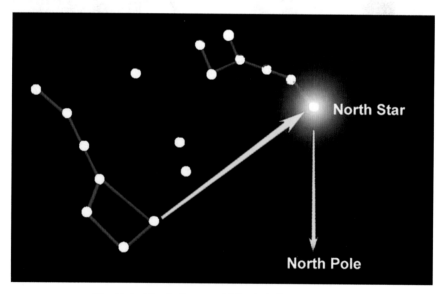

Fig. 2.4. North Star and North Pole connection

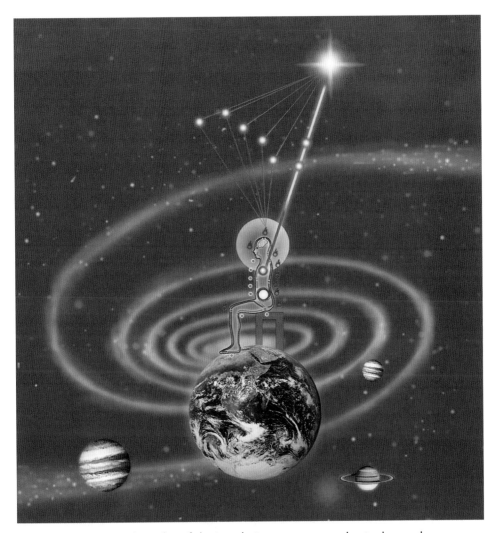

Fig. 2.5. The pulse of the North Star creates a pulse in the earth
and all its inhabitants.

ing system is established before the heart pulses. It is the North Star
that makes the earth pulse at 7.9 or nearly 8 pulses per second. In addition, the North Star is responsible for our pulse directly when we are
conceived. After the heart pulse is activated, the next one is the kidney
pulse, followed by the testicle or ovary pulse.

All together there are fifty-two pulses, but many do not function in most people. There are often a lot of blockages that need clearing. Remaining healthy is all about blood circulation and this means the pulse in different parts of the body is active. Many people are dying of blockages because their blood is not flowing properly. This is the cause of numerous illnesses because the oxygen and nutrition are not there. This frequently leads to an attack of bacteria, viruses, fungus, and mold. Health starts with the original pulse and taking care of the main organs of our bodies. Connecting with an inexhaustible pulse can extend our life. That is where the Big Dipper and North Star come in. The method is to focus on the North Star and ask it to descend so that we connect with it.

Original Pulse Method

In order to harness the power of the North Star we need to relax and allow it to descend to us. We can then feel it above our heads during its descent. Its vibration is evident and clearly recognizable if we pay attention. If the earth feels it, then most certainly we are capable of feeling it. You will feel your major organs pulse as you connect to the North Star. Ask the North Star to extend your life.

1. Sit properly in a meditative posture.
2. Send your mind's eye to the North Star.
3. Feel the pulse of the North Star.
4. This pulse initiates the other fifty-two pulses.

You need to be certain that you are connected to the North Star and the earth, moon, and sun. This is what you are connecting to and where you always reside. Human awareness is very narrow, but when connected with human consciousness it can be very wide and broad. When we connect to the Big Dipper and the North Star we receive light that is red and violet, respectively, through the Crown point (see figs. 2.6 and 2.7); we also need to connect with the golden light of the cosmic force, which we receive through the mid-eyebrow point.

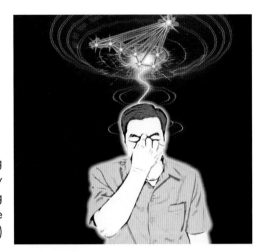

Fig. 2.6. Opening the upper mind by connecting to the Big Dipper (red light) and the North Star (violet light)

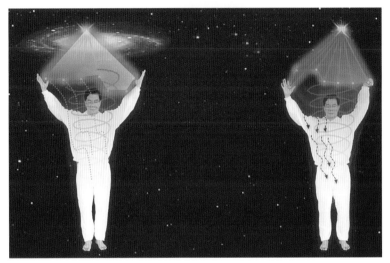

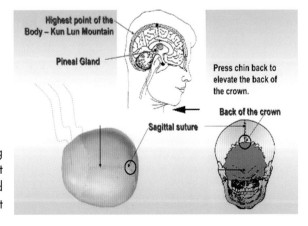

Highest point of the Body – Kun Lun Mountain

Pineal Gland

Press chin back to elevate the back of the crown.

Back of the crown

Sagittal suture

Fig. 2.7. Connecting the Crown point to the North Star and receiving the violet light

The same way that the North Star pulls a compass upward, it also pulls us upward if we are aware of it. We need to have the correct belief system to facilitate this. If we believe it, we have it. The belief system is the compass that points us in the right direction. Believing or not believing is a matter of how busy the mind is. If we are unable to believe and feel the pulse it is because we are not relaxing and letting go of the distractions in an overly busy mind. We need to relax and feel the power from above and below, but also the inward power that we have. The process is as simple as relaxing, feeling the power, and experiencing it.

Our Earth Ground

The tailbone is something like the ground wire for our connection. Just as with lightning rods, you need to have this ground or you will sustain damage when the connection strikes. The grounding needs to be complete or it is ineffective. It is just like learning how to land a plane is more important than learning how to take off or fly it. It is important to have some understanding of what we call the Dragon's Tail, the coccyx. The nerves from the brain snake and wind down the spine to the coccyx, which connect to the earth energy (see figs. 2.8 and 2.9).

All nerves in the tail are connected to the brain, and that means if

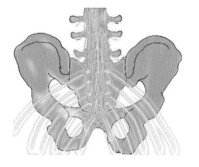

Fig. 2.8. Nerves of the coccyx and sacrum

The nerves of the coccyx and sacrum connect to twelve earthly branches of energy.

Yin–Negative Polarity Earth Energy

we move the tail we activate the entire nervous system. We must make sure to move around daily in order to get this flow activated. In the modern world we sit too much and this means that everything goes dormant (inactive). Sitting too much means the coccyx nerves do not function as well as the brain nerves. In addition, it can lead to serious and painful health issues. Being overweight and sitting too much compresses the lumbar and other parts of our nervous system and causes serious damage.

The human body has pumps located in the spine starting with the coccyx and extending up to the cranium. The anatomical pumps move back and forth, but with age they slow down and finally stop. This has a profound impact on brain function. Movement is the key to putting a stop to this problem. There is a procedure that can help prevent or slow the aging process. We start with relaxing the tailbone or coccyx

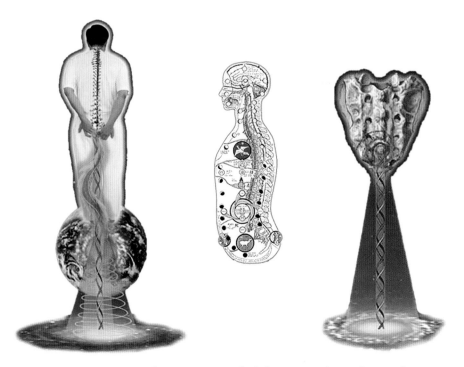

Fig. 2.9. Touch your sacrum; feel the sacrum has a long tail
extended down to the ground.

by vibrating the lower portion of the spinal column. When we move the spine in a swaying motion back and forth, all the way down to the coccyx, eventually the Fire Dragon blows fire into the coccyx by activating the spinal fluid. It then starts an upward movement, which fires the kidneys and brain, then exits the cranium and starts its energetic heavenly journey toward the North Star. When it reaches the North Star, we are pulled upward. We can actually sense the forces pulling us. The North Star is so powerful that it actually pulls the earth itself with us (see fig. 2.10).

We need to concentrate on our bodies moving upward and utilize the full strength of the North Star. We should smile toward the North Star, keeping our spine loose, flexible, and youthful. We need to align ourselves properly and lift our being and our body upward. In that fashion we are connected to the cosmos. Love, joy, and happiness are the result of connecting and transcending ourselves. When an individual

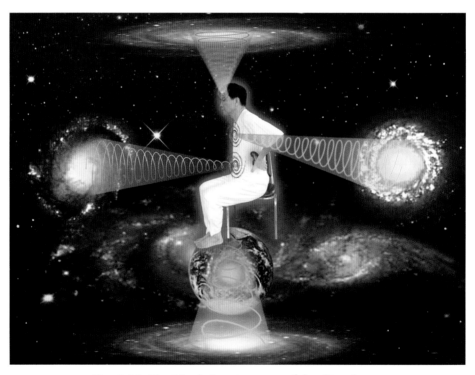

Fig. 2.10. The North Star is a powerful pulling force.

works with the North Star, they have the ability to change and adapt. This is an important survival skill. Proper alignment with the North Star is critical in attaining wisdom because it is the North Star that controls the wisdom in the solar system in which we reside.

You want to be soft and flexible because that is life. One of the secrets to all of the energetic processes that we discuss is to program the mind and body to do the practices. Program your coccyx to reach the earth and the crown to reach the North Star. After you program your being to do this, all you have to do is push the button (focus) and you will do everything correctly and dutifully.

KNOW AND LOVE YOUR ORGANS

The original operating system affects everything, including the organs in your body. These organs are vital because without them you cease to function or live. The brain is the primary receptor for new memories. While it is somewhat like a hard drive on a computer, it cannot store all of the data it receives. If it did, you would go crazy. Emotions are a different matter. They are stored in other organs such as the heart and kidneys and are a positive or negative expression of each vital organ. For example, positive emotions of kindness and generosity as well as negative emotions like anger and jealousy are generated and stored in the liver, but you are simply not aware of them. The heart holds hatred and cruelty; the spleen holds worry and anxiety; the kidneys hold fear and doubt; the lungs hold sadness and grief.

The negative emotions stored inside you are like a garbage can that has not been emptied. Even though they are stored away out of sight, they can influence you without you being aware of it. It is possible for you to get sick from these suppressed emotions, as detailed in figure 2.11, which identifies the negative emotions associated with each of the major organs, and the symptoms that can result. Anger and envy cause damage to the liver. Worry and anxiety cause damage to the stomach. Sadness and grief cause damage to the lungs and large intestine.

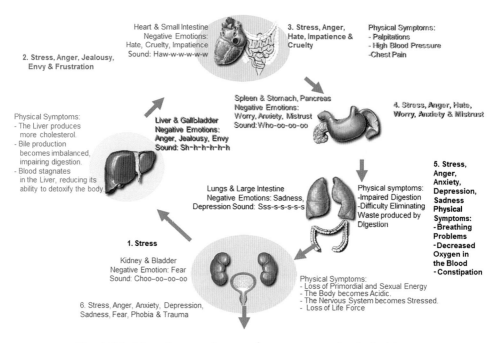

Heart & Small Intestine
Negative Emotions:
Hate, Cruelty, Impatience
Sound: Haw-w-w-w-w-w

3. Stress, Anger,
Hate, Impatience &
Cruelty

Physical Symptoms:
- Palpitations
- High Blood Pressure
- Chest Pain

2. Stress, Anger, Jealousy,
Envy & Frustration

Spleen & Stomach, Pancreas
Negative Emotions:
Worry, Anxiety, Mistrust
Sound: Who-oo-oo-oo

4. Stress, Anger, Hate,
Worry, Anxiety & Mistrust

Physical Symptoms:
- The Liver produces
  more cholesterol.
- Bile production
  becomes imbalanced,
  impairing digestion.
- Blood stagnates
  in the Liver, reducing its
  ability to detoxify the body.

Liver & Gallbladder
Negative Emotions:
Anger, Jealousy, Envy
Sound: Sh-h-h-h-h-h

5. Stress,
Anger,
Anxiety,
Depression,
Sadness
Physical
Symptoms:
- Breathing
  Problems
- Decreased
  Oxygen in
  the Blood
- Constipation

Lungs & Large Intestine
Negative Emotions: Sadness,
Depression Sound: Sss-s-s-s-s-s

Physical symptoms:
- Impaired Digestion
- Difficulty Eliminating
  Waste produced by
  Digestion

1. Stress

Kidney & Bladder
Negative Emotion: Fear
Sound: Choo-oo-oo-oo

Physical Symptoms:
- Loss of Primordial and Sexual Energy
- The Body becomes Acidic.
- The Nervous System becomes Stressed.
- Loss of Life Force

6. Stress, Anger, Anxiety, Depression,
Sadness, Fear, Phobia & Trauma

Fig. 2.11. Negative emotions and stress cause physical sickness.

Fear and doubt cause damage to the kidneys. Cruelty, indifference, and hatred cause damage to the heart.

Emotions are somewhat like garbage that can be recycled. Separating emotions is a profoundly important practice to learn and is likened to separating your garbage at home. Those who learn this are able to increase their energy rather than poison themselves. It is as simple as that. Taoists have known for thousands of years that if you have negative emotions you need to go right to the organ where they are stored, clean it out, and then clean out the link in the brain that is connected to those emotions. Then that should be followed with channeling good positive energy throughout that particular organ and the whole body.

Autonomic Nervous System

We are connected internally to a wireless universal internet that activates the autonomic nervous system, which controls action that we do not normally have to think about. It triggers either a parasympathetic or sympathetic response (see figs. 2.12 and 2.13).

A parasympathetic response signals us to "rest and digest"; it promotes digestion and calming of the nerves, and returns us to regular function. We feel love and joy or healing energy, which grows new healthy cells. The sympathetic response is triggered by fear and worry; it produces "fight or flight": defending energy for survival rather than healing. It corresponds with arousal and energy production. When we experience negative emotions or vibrations, we shut down our healing process and activate our internal army to fight or flee.

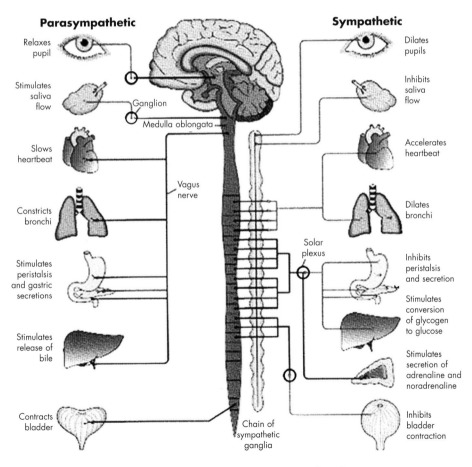

Fig. 2.12. Autonomic nervous system with either a parasympathetic or sympathetic response

The vagus nerve plays a central role in the central nervous system (see fig. 2.13). Eighty to ninety percent of the time, it reports your state of being to your brain, conveying sensory information about the state of the body's organs. If it is a sympathetic report, your kidneys will have a vasoconstriction of afferent arterioles, decreased GFR and urine volume, and your bladder will constrict the sphincter and relax the urinary bladder. If it is a parasympathetic report, your kidneys will increase urine production, your urinary bladder will tense, and the sphincter will relax to eliminate urine.

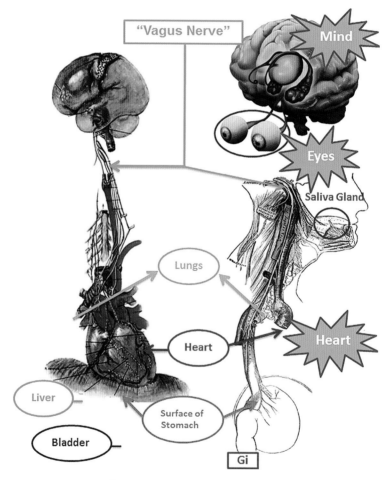

Fig. 2.13. The vagus nerve reports sensory information about the organs to the brain.

The Inner Smile

The Inner Smile is a Universal Healing Tao practice, which is actually a form of inner communication that helps you know your organs. It activates a parasympathetic response in the autonomic system, which creates (chi) energy or spiritual food (unconditional love) for our spirit and soul. The whole universe is energy and spiritual food for our spirit and soul if we can transform it.

If the reports to your brain from your body systems are always negative, your mood and actions will be negative. By always complaining you drain your life force and you are never happy. The Tao says you can look at a glass of water either half empty (negative) or half full (positive) and it is still the same glass, so you might as well look at it as half full and create a positive environment to live in. You can do this with the Inner Smile Inner Alchemy daily practice (see fig. 2.14). You can change your reports by changing the moods with a little morning

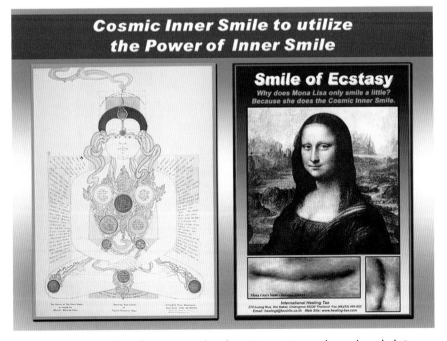

Fig. 2.14. Smile of ecstasy. Why does Mona Lisa only smile a little?
Because she does the Inner Smile.

practice each day. (Detailed instructions for a simplified version of this practice are given in chapter 4).

In the Inner Smile practice, you smile to the heart and this starts the journey to great wisdom. In this practice:

- You are defusing your negative emotions: hatred (heart), anger (liver), depression (lungs), worry (spleen), and fear (kidneys).
- You are composting negative emotions and growing positive emotions.
- You are connecting with the earth and letting go of the negative emotions into the earth.
- You are mentally going to the brain, disconnecting the negative link to the organs.
- You are then replacing the negativity with love, joy, and happiness (heart), courage and righteousness (lungs), gentleness and stillness (kidneys), kindness, generosity, and forgiveness (liver), and fairness and balance (spleen) (see fig. 2.15).

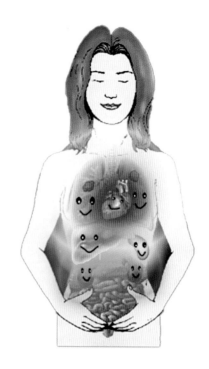

Fig. 2.15. Replacing negativity with love (heart), courage (lungs), gentleness (kidneys), kindness (liver), and balance (spleen)

In this practice, you smile to each of your inner organs. You need to know the location and appearance of your organs and trust the information that your organs transmit. When you practice visualization and proper breathing to each organ, you can experience the chi enter your being as you reach up toward the heavens and recycle the negativity into the earth. With each individual organ you start by deleting negativity. You clean everything out from time to time. That is like refreshing your computer. The more you let go, the more negativity is released from your body, spirit, and soul. The more you release to Mother Earth, the more good health and happiness will be given back to you. Do not forget to smile, not just outwardly, but inwardly too. Trust yourself even though that can be difficult. If you can trust yourself you will be able to expand your circle of existence wider and wider.

The Inner Smile practice can help you to return to your original self. However, the process is not always easy. Running through the procedure only one time will almost certainly never work. Sometimes with extreme negativity you will need weeks or even months to accomplish the cleaning out. It might take numerous times of letting go before you are cleansed totally. From a very cloudy and black mindset things will become a bright white color. You will get very healthy and you will be able to explain this to others. You will be able to help them if you are open to it.

As we have seen, the heart involves love, joy, and happiness, but also their opposites: hatred, impatience, and cruelty. The liver is similar. On the positive side are kindness and generosity and on the negative side are anger, aggressiveness, envy, jealousy, frustration, and stress. Learning how to balance emotions can lead to a life of peace and harmony, but as humans we find this difficult. However, with the Inner Smile practice, you can learn to handle your own garbage and turn it into something very positive. This means that emotions can be turned into energy.

You let all the emotional garbage go down to the earth for recycling, then you forgive, forget, and let go of depression, anger, and regret. After you release the negative data in your organs, it is vital to disconnect the link that still remains in your mind. This is a relatively easy process, somewhat like operating a computer. By looking up to your brain and rocking side to side as you look from your left brain to right brain a number of times, your mind will be cleaned out. It will disconnect the negative links and you will have fresh memories of love, joy, happiness, courage, and righteousness. By doing this daily you will be in control of your emotions and you will face the day with a positive attitude.

If you have your priorities right you realize that good health is the best investment of all. Some sicknesses are incurable; money cannot buy your way out. There is no escape. If you are busy making money at the expense of your health, it is a bad investment of your time. While it is true that sometimes you are busy, at least you have time to activate the Inner Smile and make a connection to your Original Source or God. It can become a way of life as well as a lifelong healthy habit (see fig. 2.16).

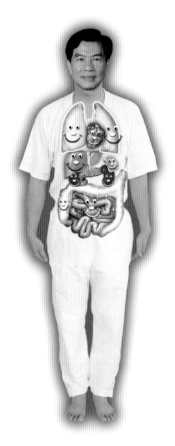

Fig. 2.16. Smiling to your heart and other organs to bring about positive energy is something you can easily activate even if you are busy.

Unlimited Love

All religions want to connect to God and people want to have God within them. When you have negativity in the form of anger, jealousy, hatred, and forms of discord, you shut off this connection. This connection is necessary in order to receive the gift of unconditional, unlimited, and universal love. The Original Spirit in the heart connects to the Supreme Creator, which activates the love, joy, and happiness in your heart.

Understand the theory and practice it: turn to your own being to find love, joy, and happiness so you can spread that sensation to your entire body and the environment that is your home. You were born to be connected, so you link yourself to the Supreme Creator in whatever form you envision that aligns with your personal belief system. Your heart is activated; this is followed by the violet light. The wisdom that is your destiny will then be easily accessible to you.

The love that you have is finite and limited, but if you avail yourself of cosmic unlimited love, your own love can multiply. If you want to find love, it is pointless to go around the world looking for it in others. Love is within your own heart and being. The heart is where you store love, joy, and happiness. You are responsible for the experience of love and will never find it externally. You are unable to help others if you have negativity within yourself. If you have hatred in your heart, there is no way you can assist those you meet on your journey through life. A compassionate life is a life lived well and with purpose.

The Tao finds that in balance, and part of such balance is to turn outward as well as inward. If you have love in your heart, it radiates out to other organs. Then it radiates out from your organs to other people and all your surroundings. This starts with loving yourself and then loving those that you can love. That kind of love expands because it is real.

Calming the Monkey Mind

The Taoists call our mind the monkey mind because it gets us into a lot of monkey business or busy activities that are unimportant. There are many ways to quiet a mind that thinks too much. A mantra is one way; focusing on symbols or statues is another, and there are numerous other methods. The important thing is whether they help you to change your thinking and still your monkey mind.

The best way to keep the monkey mind focused is to train it (see fig. 2.17). They actually have a monkey school in Thailand where monkeys are trained to gather coconuts. They even know when to pick coconuts that are ripe. In the case of humans, the monkey mind moves and it is actually impossible to empty it completely. The type of meditation that teaches emptying of the mind is not the right path for many people. When you are healthy you have energy, and when you have energy you move. The issue is where you move and what you do. If you use the energy to train yourself correctly then you will have a meaningful, happy, and productive life. That is what the Tao teaches us.

This is a big task but the internal active meditations of the Universal Healing Tao system work, when done daily for just five to ten minutes. The Inner Smile method is the best for many because it entails looking at your organs and creating a nice, warm feeling. Your mind then

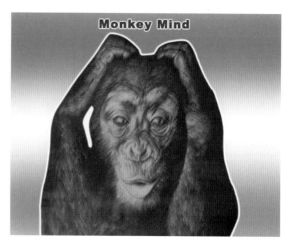

Fig. 2.17. Train your monkey mind so that you do not waste your chi.

focuses on that good feeling and the monkey stops jumping around. This is what is termed energetic or moving meditation.

EMPOWERING YOURSELF

Initially, when you focus on something, you send energy to it. If one million people focus on a single individual, they give that person a lot of power. No matter what you are focused on, you are giving it power. You need to keep in mind this important factor. If a system, movement, or church gets bigger and bigger, you get smaller and smaller because the power of the movement is growing with the number of people involved. In this Taoist system you are focused on yourself. You are not giving your power away. You empower yourself by strengthening your organs.

When you go in search of your soul or spirit, it is easy to recognize it when you find it. Simply look at the various organs and their colors. Your body is the temple that matters. Your soul and spirit live there. Each organ has its own palace and its own special color. The heart, which contains the Original Spirit, is red. If you want to be in touch with your Original Spirit, you go into your heart. The different aspects of your being can be found in the different organs of your body.

The green Hun soul is stored in the liver and is in charge of thinking, planning, dreaming, and other mysterious things. The spleen holds the power of intention. The pure soul, which is white, is involved in all kinds of emotional aspects and is stored in the lungs. Blue willpower is stored in the kidneys. At this initial stage of your search, it is critical that you get in contact with your energy.

Charging the Human Bio-Battery

While humans are limited, they are bioelectric creatures and have the ability to channel energy. There is a very simple rule and that is that you should tap into the available energy surrounding you. A living cell can store energy, and the more energy you have the more you can store.

If you do not do that you will exhaust all your own energy and it will eventually be totally depleted. This is the teaching of the Taoist masters of old, and there is no need to reinvent the wheel. All you need to do is ask for the force and the door will open.

To make sure that you have sufficient energy means that you keep your battery charged. You need to recharge your batteries with sleep, food, and positive emotional energy stored in the lower tan tien. You need to be very conscientious about working your tan tien because maintaining a charge is critical to your life. If your battery does not work, you cannot have life. You are, in essence, like an expensive car with a dead battery. Similarly, you do not want to walk around in a daze with little or no energy. Unfortunately we see more and more people in this condition nowadays walking around in a state of chronic fatigue. There are people who are always in this unfortunate state because they have failed to recharge their personal battery.

Some people believe that they need to send energy out to the universe. This is misguided because the universe is not in need of your energy; it has enough of its own. Energy needs to be stored and recharged, not foolishly sent out into the universe or wasted on lost causes. You need to take advantage of the fact that your body has the ability to recharge itself, because it can diminish over time.

When our natural battery runs low, the forces in our body that fight disease and depression are unable to function. We should recharge our bodies daily by utilizing the plug that nature gave us to connect us to the universe: the navel. This plug can be charged by placing the middle finger from each hand directly into the navel and mentally drawing energy into the lower tan tien. You will feel the abdomen getting warmer and warmer as it is recharged; then your kidneys will start getting warmer in your lower back. The first sign that you are recharging your battery 60 to 70 percent is that you do not get sick.

We can use the energy of the universe to recharge our own personal battery. In order to activate our crown and kidney power, we can rub our hands together in front of our face and then ask for the pulse of the North Star. As we extend our hands, we will feel the pulse. Next we need to consider our kidneys. The brain has nerves that connect to the kidneys and the heart has blood vessels that are connected. We put our mind, our eyes, and the heart together and look into the kidneys. When ready, we exhale and hold our breath until we need to breathe. Then, as we breathe normally, each breath should be felt moving into the kidneys. Our breath becomes balanced and the kidneys get warmer. Our life will then begin to change because our organs are getting the proper oxygen.

If we can hold our breath without panicking then we can relax properly. Chi enters our kidneys when we do this. We continue this until we feel our stomach pulling in and our testicles or ovaries going down. Everything is pulsing together. With each breath we feel the kidneys pulsing. Eventually the stomach creates suction and pulls the ovaries or testicles upward with each breath. This facilitates a connection to the brain because your lower brain (in the stomach) is connected to your upper brain (in your head). Finally every breath is connected to the kidneys, brain, and testicles or ovaries. The goal is to get four diaphragms moving. The urogenital diaphragm and the pelvic diaphragm are connected to the brain diaphragm (see fig. 2.18).

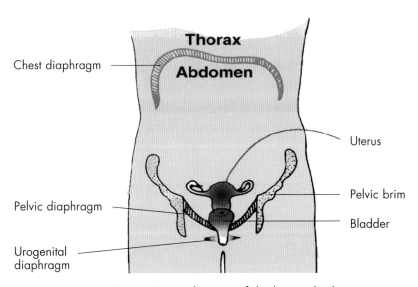

Fig. 2.18. Diaphragms of the human body

Your Personal Power Generator

Everyone has forces around them that are spinning in different directions. The forces that are spinning external to your being activate the forces inside you. The internal forces are your chi. In total there are four forces, all going in different ways (see fig. 2.19). Awareness of these forces and the spinning provides us with what amounts to a free ride.

The only thing that you need to be sure of is that those forces

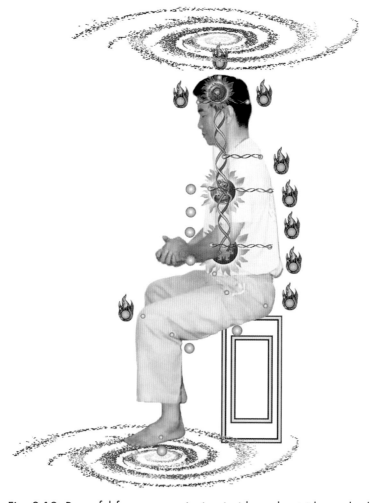

Fig. 2.19. Powerful forces are spinning inside and outside our body.

are gyrating in different directions inside you. The sum total of this is your own personal power generator, your electric power plant (see fig. 2.20).

You have four Tai Chi balls spinning in different directions, which generate all of your power. To understand the four Tai Chi symbols, you need to remember the fact that the yin and yang symbol is spinning: if you examine it carefully, you can see that yin and yang are rotating.

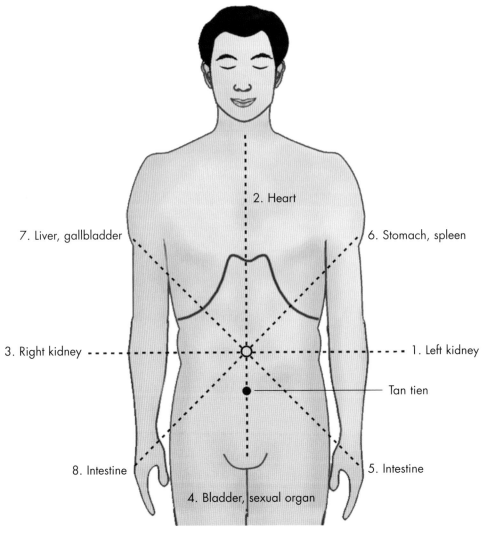

Fig. 2.20. The generator is in the area of the navel.

Yin pushes yang and yang pushes yin. Yin and yang are interdependent: nothing wins and nothing loses. With the spinning of the four Tai Chi balls, a chi ball develops at the core of our being and in the center of our body. The chi ball is spinning inside us like the earth spinning around itself (see fig. 2.21).

The spinning of the four Tai Chi balls generates power. You are born with this ability to produce power. No one can give that to you because you already have it, just like you have a spirit that is immortal. You have the power to move the chi ball, but the four Tai Chi balls do not move (although they do spin). The area in the lower abdomen where the four yin yang symbols spin is a very important area for all practitioners of the Tao, known as the Hua Hin (see fig. 2.22).

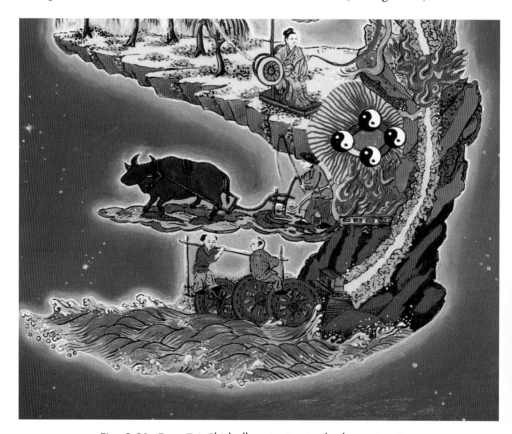

Fig. 2.21. Four Tai Chi balls spinning in the lower tan tien
creating a chi ball

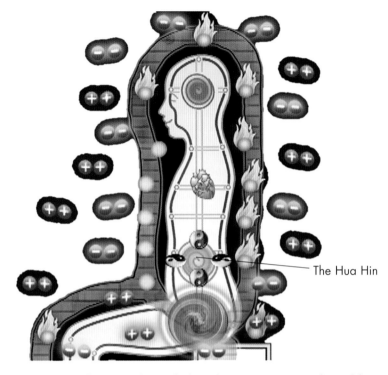

The Hua Hin

Fig. 2.22. The four Tai Chi symbols within you create inexhaustible energy as they rotate in what is known as the Hua Hin area.

Being aware of and utilizing the Hua Hin creates a chi ball that transmits energy to the sexual organs. You create the chi ball as a container for your energy so that you can draw on it when you need it. Eventually you can develop your own chi ball to the place where it condenses into a pearl that holds everything that is important in your universe. Indeed it is your own personal universe. After you discover you can capture chi in a ball, you can utilize it. You simply need to trust, focus, and concentrate. The result is a unification of your natural-born internal fire, which is energy. You should make this process a part of your daily life so it is like the eternally refilling well.

Taoism is not nearly as mysterious as most religions. It does not involve all kinds of magic. Actually, considering how far it dates back, it is quite scientific, and science has verified many of the theories of ancient Taoism. While some of the Taoist language is metaphorical, there are clearly specific scientific equivalents of the vocabulary involved. Keeping this in mind, you need to understand what the Taoist masters meant when they talked about your "well." By this they were referring to a gathering point within you; a place for the storage of your energy.

Suppose you dig a hole in the ground. Clearly the result is that water will fill the hole up. Using this concept, the next step is to acknowledge the well within you. Just like a well in the ground continues to fill with water, so too does the sexual orgasmic energy within you have a gathering place.

The Million Dollar Point

In the perineum area there is a mysterious point. In the olden days this was termed a point worth a thousand pieces of gold or roughly a million dollars, which is the origin of the term "Million Dollar point." In ancient times, anatomy was not a subject that was widely known or studied. The Taoist masters were among the few who knew of the great mystery of life and its relationship to human anatomy. The ancients would have a Taoist master come into the royal court and make sure to close the seven doors. The Taoist apprentices would remove their trousers and the master would touch the Million Dollar point for them. The million dollars was the price for being shown where the point is. If the Taoist student did not get it, then they would never understand the mysteries of the universe.

The Hui Yin, the "place where the yin gathers," is the point that is the center of the mystery. The yin energy is like oil and when the Hui Yin is activated, it opens and all the energy flows in. The point is the center of energy and at the same time the place where you are grounded to the earth. You can also think of it as the perineum area (see fig. 2.23).

The Hui Yin is located between the sexual organs and the anus

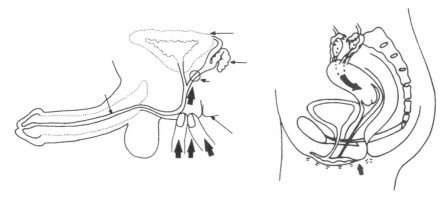

Fig. 2.23. The Hui Yin is located in the part of the body called the perineum.

(see fig. 2.24). This area is often called the Gate of Life and Death, with the sexual organ being the seat of life and the anus being the seat of death. The anus is the area where energy is released. Energy leakage can shorten your life. It is possible to gather and hold energy in the Hui Yin. If you put the oil you have gathered onto a fire, the fire burns longer; this is equivalent to adding life. This is essentially the mystery of sexual Taoism.

It is very important for you to remember that in the region under discussion there are crossroads. Above you connect to the crown;

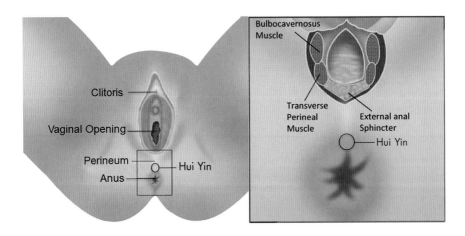

Fig. 2.24. The true Hui Yin point is in front of the anus.

below and in front you connect to the soles and the feet connect to the earth. In front it connects to your sexual organs, and in back to your anus.

If you massage the Million Dollar point every day, you will feel it relaxing and energy gathering. You begin with finding the spot just in front of your anus where your middle finger can go in about one inch. After you locate this place you can connect it to the crown by inhaling, contracting it, and rolling your eyes up. Then you exhale and release. A few repetitions followed by relaxation will bring about a gathering of all the yin energy.

The Microcosmic Orbit Meditation

As mentioned earlier, spinning is the nature of the universe. Both in a macrocosmic and microcosmic sense, there is movement. The various planets, solar systems, and galaxies all have their own orbits. This is true on a smaller scale as well. Within the cells of your body electrons orbit around the nucleic protons and neutrons. You can actually feel the earth spinning as well as the sun and moon. You not only feel macrocosmic orbits but microcosmic orbits as well (see fig. 2.25). The patterns for these orbits are very similar and they all generate power or electricity. These orbits are eternal, and it is possible for us to tap into their nature.

From the microcosmic perspective, the better the electrons and neutrons spin, the more chi you have and consequently the healthier you are. The thing to recognize is that the movement and orbits of your life in a very real sense actually are your life. They are you. The Microcosmic Orbit exercise can be used to implement the power of orbits in your life. Detailed instructions are given in chapter 4.

In the Microcosmic Orbit exercise, you sit and rock your spine, which starts to connect with the Heavens (positive charge: yang) and Earth (negative charge: yin). You energetically extend your tailbone or Dragon's Tail into the earth's energy field and ground yourself in

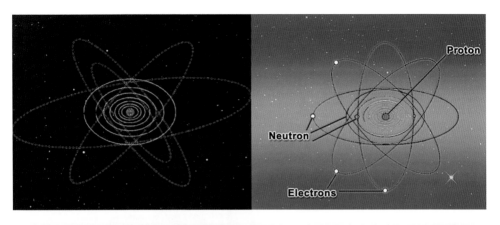

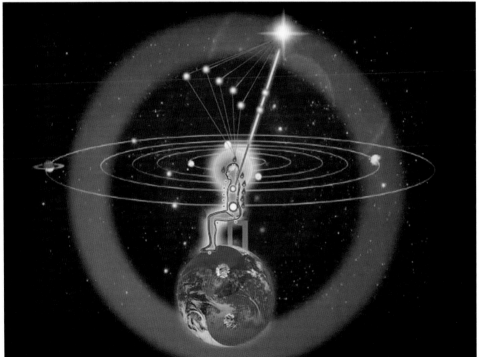

Fig. 2.25. Macrocosmic and microcosmic orbits

the earth. You will feel your coccyx getting very long as you relax and vibrate it into the earth. As you relax and absorb the earth energy into your body, you will feel the Fire Dragon come up into your spinal cord, activating all your organs (see fig. 2.26 on page 80).

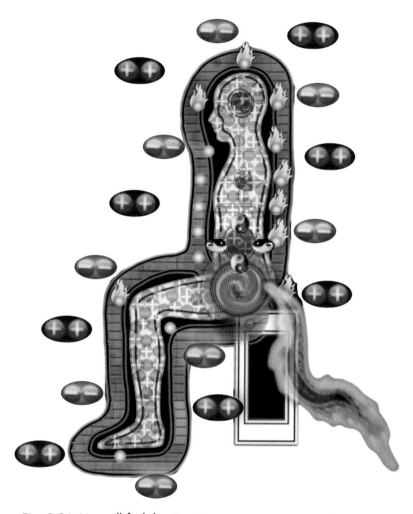

Fig. 2.26. You will feel the Fire Dragon surge up your spine to
your crown as you tap into Mother Earth.

This practice will also tune you in to your local connection to the
cosmos, which is just above your head, drawing intelligence, wisdom,
and unconditional love from the North Star (violet light) into your
heart, crown, and lower tan tien (see fig. 2.27). The heart acts as a wireless receiver to draw down the violet light of unconditional love, which
feeds the body organs and connects to sexual orgasmic energy.

The connection above and below will activate the four Tai Chi balls

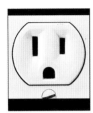

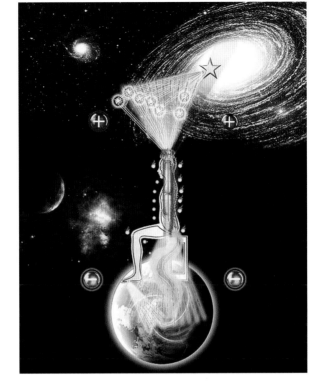

Fig. 2.27. Wired into the pulsation of the North Star

at the lower tan tien, which will begin spinning in different directions. The four spinning aspects of our being become a fireball that drops to the sexual organs and provides sexual energy. This procedure is necessary in order to produce any transformation or alchemy.

As you spin your energy, it starts to balance itself, whereas prior to that it was unbalanced. You will create much more energy for yourself. You will be able to feel the energetic fire flowing into the sexual organs. The sexual energy that is produced in this fashion is like a ball of fire torching a stack of wood. There is fire and the fire is energy. This energy is called the Almighty One. The name derives from the ability of sexual energy to create life. Your very existence is the result of the Almighty One.

Earth energy also is activated and it then begins to travel up to your heart. It transforms to spiritual energy. The Original Spirit is the leader and the spiritual food comes together in the heart. Unbelievable happiness is now possible and you will be able to be born again in a new life. The main thing is that you know and feel it yourself. You are your own witness. No one else can make you know it, just as no one can make you know anything. The knowledge is subjective and only in that way does it lead to your own certainty. You will know clearly that something inside you has transformed.

Simple Energy Activation

There are some very simple things you can do to activate your energy. You can rub your hands together to make them warm and proceed to rub your face with them. Go all the way to your ears. Rub your hands together again and then cover your eyes. You will feel the heat. The eyes contain chi and have very small capillaries. We must be sure that there is no blockage in the eyes. The procedure for the eyes is to first close them and use the hands in unison to gently sweep outward. This is done very lightly. It will get the blood flowing in the eyes. This should be done 18 or 36 times. Next, we close the eyes one at a time and rub them with the soft portion of the fingertips, *very* lightly. If there is pain with this gentle rubbing, that is actually good; it will stop after a period of time. This also gets the blood flowing and can assist with migraine headaches.

Following this, click your teeth together several times. The teeth have important nerves that go directly to the brain. By strengthening the gums and the teeth we can tap into additional energy in our bodies. Clicking our teeth together lightly activates the nerves and lets energy flow to the brain (see fig. 2.28). This additional energy can be used, for example, if we are driving and feel sleepy. By simply clicking the teeth together, we can feel the energy flow and be rejuvenated. What is taking place in such cases is that we are fooling the kidneys in order to get the additional energy. This should be done with caution; if we do it too much we will deplete the reserve energy and have none for those

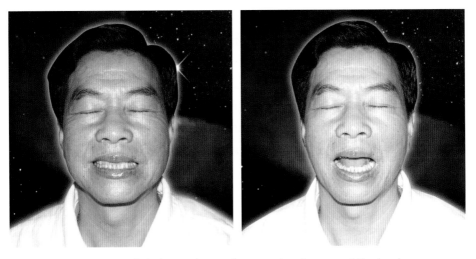

Fig. 2.28. Click the teeth together evenly—front, middle, back.

times where we require it, such as when we are sick or exhausted. This reserve energy can save our lives and should not be used without seriously considering what we are doing.

The next step is to rotate the tongue in the mouth so that the salivary gland is activated. Following this we eat the cosmos as the air mixes with the saliva. The saliva holds a lot of oxygen and nitrogen. The process of eating and chewing the air transforms it into liquid oxygen and liquid nitrogen. After mixing this together well in the mouth, we then swallow the saliva by locking the neck. We do this several times as we swallow hard and rub the navel.

The ears come next. They are covered with the hands, with the fingers pointing back. The ears are covered and then opened several times. In the back of the head in a line directly behind the ears is the mechanical portion of the ears. Keeping both hands over the ears and tapping the back of the head with the fingers helps us maintain our balance. Hit the back of your head with an open hand. You can softly hit your ears. Using the fingertips, rub around your ears.

You will have a warm sensation and arousal that might be near an orgasm. Energy from the earth, your crown, and the heavens gathers in the Hui Yin. You want this energy to move upward to your lower tan tien. Breathe properly, moving the energy up to your Door of Life (see fig. 2.29). Remember all things in the cosmos are connected. You must only trust and then activate. Healing will take place.

Following this, hit the middle of the chest with your fist and then laugh out loud, which activates your thymus and then your abdomen. You simply slap it and laugh out loud. When there is no gas or other blockages, blood can flow and you are actually creating antibodies. Use a similar technique with your liver, spleen, and even your legs. These exercises are ones that add life force into your life because there is more Original Chi. Taoist practices like this are thousands of years old and ultimately entail transforming sexual energy into spiritual energy.

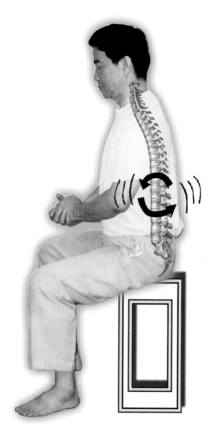

Fig. 2.29. Feel the warmth in your Door of Life.

Chi Self-Massage

Chi Self-Massage is based on the fact that the energy of the body moves through a series of channels that travel from your vital organs to the surface of your skin. These channels (meridians, acupuncture points, and nerve endings) are the communications network of your body—like the electrical wiring in your house. The paths can become blocked from inside the organs or within the network itself, resulting in malfunction.

Living in our unnatural environments puts a lot of stress on our bodies. We all need a simple technique for releasing built-up stress and the blockages it can cause. By simply touching the extremities (skin) of your body, you can connect daily to your vital organs and open up any blockages within the network. When you massage your face, neck, chest, hands, arms, legs, and feet you release stress and tension from the whole system. By applying Chi Self-Massage formulas after daily practice, after any long sitting or standing period, or any time you feel tension throughout the day, you can literally keep in touch with yourself, opening the body and the vital organs as needed. Detailed instructions are given in chapter 4.

Cooling Your Energy with Six Healing Sounds

You are driving your car down the street and on your dashboard the red temperature light goes on. If you do not stop the car and check the engine, what happens? The car's engine will explode, because it has overheated. Your body has a cooling system similar to that of your car. The connective tissue (fascia) around your vital organs absorbs any excess heat and releases it through your skin and digestive tract. When you urinate, defecate, yawn, belch, or sweat you release heat. If the release is blocked through years of improper diet and lack of exercise, the vital organs will explode or stop functioning; you may have a heart attack, impaired kidneys, or liver malfunction because your body's cooling system has broken down and the vital organs have become overheated. The

Six Healing Sounds formula activates your cooling system on a daily basis by restructuring the connective tissue to function properly around your vital organs; its postures result in cooling them down by releasing the condensed heat with their individual sounds. In the practice of the Six Healing Sounds, you breathe in slowly, aware of each of your vital organs in turn, then breathe out any negative emotions associated with that organ, while making the appropriate sound (see fig. 2.30).

SIX HEALING SOUNDS

The lungs' sound: sss-s-s-s-s

The kidneys' sound: choo-oo-oo-oo

The liver's sound: sh-h-h-h-h

The heart's sound: haw-w-w-w-w-w

The spleen's sound: who-oo-oo-oo

The triple warmer's (or heater's) sound: hee-e-e-e-e

Detailed instructions can be found in chapter 4.

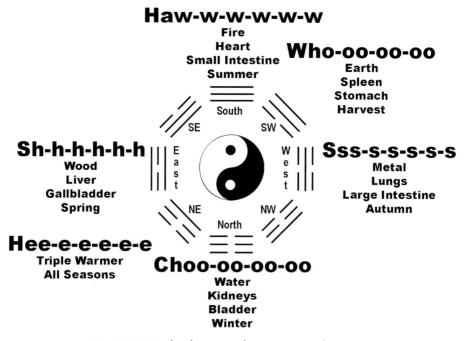

Fig. 2.30. Six healing sounds, organs, and seasons

TAOIST SECRETS OF TRANSFORMING SEXUAL ENERGY

Much of the modern world is fixated on sex, but the approach is generally wrong-minded and leaves people still desiring true satisfaction. They want a more meaningful life, but unfortunately they often waste their life away in pointless unproductive fun and miss out on the true purpose of their existence. Businesses take advantage of this with an endless procession of sexual titillation in the form of advertising while at the same time the pornography market floods the internet. There is nothing wrong with pornography per se; the problem lies with the waste of sexual energy that is necessary for life. The purpose of sexual arousal is not simply to have an orgasm but to have an orgasm that you can hold in the organs and transform into energy. This transformation is crucial because attaining the higher level of orgasm permits you to attain pure happiness.

Love and a meaningful orgasm are not separable. Merely to ejaculate is not just a waste of time but a waste of chi. With loving sex two forces become one and everything in your life is happier. It takes some time to come to this simple realization, but once attained it will transform your life. The basic energy for everyone is love, arousal, and orgasm as a united force that becomes one transformative Primordial Force. When the human body is formed, the sexual organs and the kidneys store part of the Ching Chi, the essence of the Primordial Force. The heart stores part of the Original Spirit (Yuan Shen) of the Primordial Force.

When we combine our love, compassion, and orgasmic sexual energy, a harmonizing resonance effect arises at the synergistic frequency of eight hertz. In this state of activation, our cells will draw in the Primordial Force and a process of cellular intercourse occurs. DNA is transcribed in the nucleus and translated from RNA in the cytoplasm. Cells divide and combine, giving birth to new and improved cells. This cellular intercourse will also occur when enough of this combined sexual energy is stored and then combined with love and compassion energy. Thus, we can give our new cells' DNA the support of the creative life forces that nurtured our first cell—original reproductions, but genetically-enhanced versions through the power of "positive personal engineering."

To progress with the practice of the Tao we need to understand the notion of sexual energy on a very high level. Refraining from sex is frequently one aspect of the way some seekers strive for a higher state of being. This is evidenced by the fact that priests, nuns, monks, and other holy men or holy women are celibate. One might conclude from this that those who do have sexual intercourse are not holy, even though they have sex when married. This can also be interpreted as sexual energy being the key to communicating with a higher power.

The reason all the great traditions emphasize celibacy is because sex involves losing something. However, this does not mean that transcendence entails not utilizing sexual energy. In addition, scientific reports have highlighted the fact that celibacy can create problems associated with prostate cancer, uterine cancer, and breast cancer. It is similar to the familiar saying "if you do not use it, you lose it." When an infant breastfeeds this is of great benefit to a woman, showing us, among other things, that simply not using our organs is not the way to approach transcendence.

Whether you are a man or a woman, you are probably just throwing away energy. Most men, for the majority of their life, simply waste their sexual energy in genital orgasms. For women, the energy is often trapped in their breasts and is hurting them. Next, all of the energy reserved for the egg to make a baby is simply flushed out every month. Taoists have taught for centuries that this throwing away of energy is a terrible waste, which causes you to get old and sick and die. The good news is that you can take it back. When you take it back it becomes the original forces, which you can use as spiritual food. You can give this food to your soul and spirit. You will then be doing something for both this life and your next life. You can accumulate spiritual credit that helps you now and helps you later. No one can steal this because it goes only to your soul and spirit.

The ancient Taoist masters knew of the benefits of utilizing sexual energy thousands of years ago. Sexual energy can be used to the benefit of health, longevity, and happiness. Many of the techniques that are used by the Chinese Taoist masters have their origins in India. The Taoists adopted numerous secrets of ancient India. The secrets of the Taoist masters were passed down orally at first and always utilized sexual techniques that recognized the inner power available to everyone. The Living Tao Sexual Alchemy practices are ways to transform sexual energy into life force and then to spirit force. They include male and female practices for Single and Dual Cultivation (see fig. 2.31). Detailed instructions are given in chapter 5, "Sexual Alchemy."

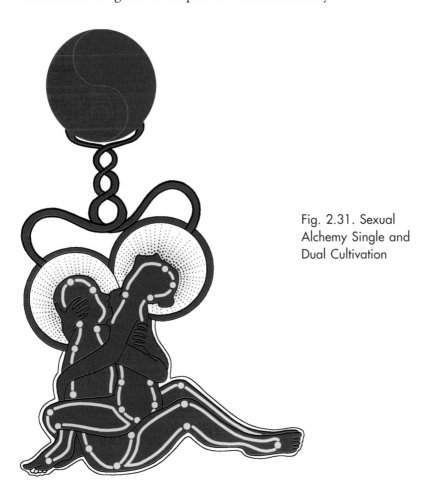

Fig. 2.31. Sexual Alchemy Single and Dual Cultivation

Being an Immortal

Everyone knows that it is critical to see no evil, hear no evil, and speak no evil. What that should actually mean is that we do not see such things in others. See the goodness in people and concentrate on that. One method of doing that is to use a Tibetan skull cup. This is a cup made from an actual human skull, used for rituals by Tibetan monks. Frequently they are elaborately carved and have a covering of precious metals and jewels. Many have openings where the chi was received and the energy connected to the North Star and beyond. For the true student the opening at the top of the skull is literally there.

The Way of the Tao is simple but practicing it is not easy. Once you recognize the simplicity of the Taoist practice, you are then wise, because ultimate wisdom and truth is obvious and clear to you. You were born to be an immortal. The question is what kind of immortal you will be. Sexual energy is the only type of energy that can be transformed and is the path toward immortality. While energy can be neither created nor destroyed, it can be transformed and flow from one place to another.

Intercourse is not something that happens just between humans. You can have intercourse with your own mind and spirit or with the gods and goddesses. This opens you up to the violet light, which is an intelligent force. You do not want to leave this world with a child spirit or as a hungry ghost. Educate yourself and know what the purpose of your life is. Avoid ignorance and seek wisdom. You cannot buy rank or prestige in the next life. Wisdom leading to enlightenment is the key. Incorporate the practices of the Tao, and a meaningful life is virtually guaranteed. The universe is multidimensional in nature and is made up of the polar energies of yin and yang. These are a fundamental nondual unity that we grasp by having wisdom and practicing sexual cultivation.

True and meaningful intercourse actually does make love; it creates it, and from love everything comes forward. True unity and transcendence is possible only through making love, which is to say, true and meaningful sexual intercourse. Such intercourse can be partaken of utilizing different methods.

Turning the Senses Inward

In the Taoist tradition, when you turn inward, you can grasp the real point of the senses and the purpose of sensuality. Bodily understanding is one of the most important doors to open in order to grasp eternity.

The Tao teaches us that

- The eyes are the window of the liver.
- The ears are the window of the kidneys.
- The tongue is the window of the heart.
- The mouth is the window of the spleen.
- The nose is the window of the lungs.

These windows can be opened as well as closed. In the practice of the Tao the windows do not have to be completely shut or completely open. Intelligence needs to be used with any window because it involves energy. If you keep a window of your house open in the middle of winter, the result may be that you freeze to death. At the very least it can mean you lose the heat from your furnace, which can cost you a lot of money and waste energy.

The windows to your organs are also windows to your soul and your spirit. They need proper monitoring. You can practice what monkeys do and cover your eyes, cover your ears, and cover your mouth. You can even cover your sexual organs and do no evil. The next step is to turn your senses inward and pay attention to your inner body. This involves totally perceiving your major inner organs by utilizing your ears, eyes, and mouth to make this critical connection.

To start you can turn your ears inward and hear the music and harmony of your body. Hear the waterfall, the mountain stream, and the beautiful music that is coming from your kidneys. You will hear many sounds in each and every part of your body, but the ears should relate particularly to your kidneys. The sounds are natural and cosmic in the way they come forth.

Surrender your senses to God or the Ultimate, or whatever name you have chosen to relate to the most powerful source in the cosmos. Match it with your own personal belief system. Give yourself permission to see the Prime Mover while making sure to concentrate on the goodness of all things positive. Take particular note of seeing the goodness of other people and all sentient beings. It is far better to see goodness, because perceiving evil and negativity drains you of your life force. Sometimes this is difficult to do because we live in a world filled with negativity of rivalries, hatred, envy, and greed. All you have to do is watch the news to know how much we are surrounded by negative forces. The Tao says that no matter how bad something is, there is always a good side. This is quite clear in the concept of yin and yang. Everything negative is counterbalanced by the positive. If it is possible for you to see the good, then it is possible for you to grow and add significance to all of the aspects of your worldview. Doing so facilitates energy to assist you in your journey.

One way to do this is to connect your tongue down to your heart. Your tongue is used for speech, which is essential for communication, for connecting with other people. When you want to say something, especially something important, always think three times. Thinking and speech have a very close relationship and ultimately are a major factor in determining who you are and who you become. Keep in mind that your being is constantly changing as you speak, act, and interact with the world. To be a person of character, the tongue must be pure.

In the same fashion as you turned your ears toward your kidneys, turn your eyes toward the liver. Turn your nose toward the lungs. Turn your mouth toward the spleen. Listen for and hear the music of nature and all living things. Smile and breathe and open yourself up to the life forces of Mother Earth and the violet light of enlightenment. Know

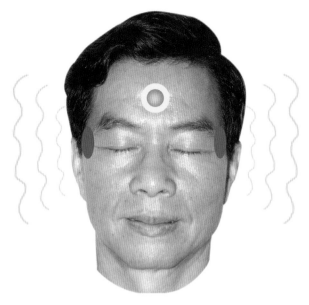

Fig. 2.32. Turning your senses inward helps you find
your love, joy, and happiness.

yourself. In this fashion, everything turns toward the center of your being (see fig. 2.32).

Turning your senses inward is a step in the process of finding not only happiness but your true being. Mere sensual gratification is very limited in terms of personal fulfillment. Your inner world is always available to you and can, in a sense, contain more metaphysical stability than the external world. Your inner being never goes away. It is truly something that is impossible to lose. You can know safety, security, and happiness subjectively to a greater degree than you can know it objectively. Simply relax, let go, breathe, and feel the corresponding autonomy that the cosmos provides.

FUSION

One of the most important things to remember is chi comes and chi goes. This necessitates learning a process capable of containing and transforming chi. The mind, soul, spirit, eyes, and other sensory organs are capable, with practice, of containing chi in a chi ball or pearl. This means that chi can be fixed or stabilized. The first thing is the mind and second is saliva. If you can fix chi in water you can contain it. After that you can fix it into something more solid. This is Taoist Fusion practice. Once you fix the pearl it contains power. This alchemical process is one of the secrets of the great Taoist masters.

The entire practice of the Tao involves invoking the primordial forces to reunite with your body, but it has a flexible and open-minded approach to everything. No matter where we are, we are well positioned for the important process of utilizing the primordial forces of life. The Taoist masters have taught us that the universe provides energy to our being and to the earth. The earth's function is to support life and it is wise for us to keep that in mind.

The sexual organs are the inexhaustible well of your personal energy. You need to learn to cultivate, control, conserve, refine, and store your sexual energy in the body as part of your own spiritual quest. When you do the Taoist practices, your body and mind are continuously refreshed and replenished.

The first thing that happens when you start the Fusion practices is that the energy goes up to your brain and activates your pituitary gland, the thalamus, hypothalamus, and pineal gland. The energy then begins to flow into your mouth. At this point you gather your energy in the Hui Yin and blend every source of energy into one single force. Generating sexual energy in this manner is an essential part of your spiritual development. When done properly the sexual energy is drawn upward from the genitals to the lower tan tien to create an internal energizing fire of power and energy (see fig. 2.33).

In the Fusion practices, four eight-sided pakuas are created and used to draw the organs' energies into their spinning centers. The pakua symbol has representations of the eight forces corresponding to the Eight Immortals. The center is composed of the Tai Chi symbol of yin and yang entwining.

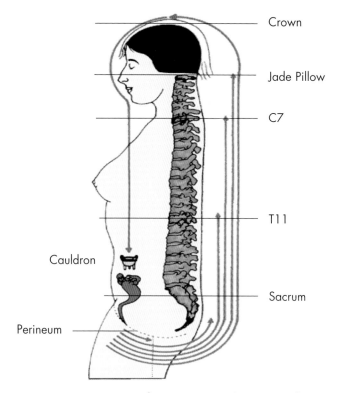

Fig. 2.33. Draw sexual energy upward to create chi.

The Fusion practices are dependent on interaction with your internal organs. They are a way of composting negative energy from all of the organs. Through the Fusion processes, the organs' energy is transformed and any negative emotional qualities or imbalances from the organs are neutralized. The transformed energy becomes more refined and balanced, stronger and attuned to a higher quality. Then it can be brought back as a positive force to the pakuas, which function as a transformational resource. There is then a blending stage where positive energy forms as a result of communicating with the organs and the energy of the cosmos.

The more you practice this, the easier it will become. Your health will benefit and negativity will dissipate. You will be more energetically advanced. When the four pakuas are activated, they begin spinning.

You will feel this in a very noticeable fashion. The image is similar to that of the planets circling the sun, which can make you feel like you are the center of the universe. In a sense, perhaps more personal than factual, you *are* the center of the universe. You can sense the energy of the forces around you. If you pay attention, visualize, and fine-tune your sense of sight, you will see this taking place. The four pakuas form a shield around you that protects you from negativity.

You must also recognize the pull of the North Star and Southern Cross. When you gather this energy in your being, there is a direct connection to your axis that extends to these all-powerful stars. It reaches out to the other planets and their moons. Eventually you have something like a wifi connection that extends to the universe and you are able to download knowledge.

Fusion involves knowledge of the solar system. If you have no understanding of this it will only lead to con-fusion, not Fusion itself. Know the planets and how they spin. Realize that in every rotation there is always an axis. Human beings are given a brain and two hands. With these, you should be able to stay balanced, focused, and aligned. It is possible with study and practice to use the energy of the solar system to bring forth the cosmic and earth forces that can empower and protect you. In this way your internal organs permit your life force to ultimately connect once again to the stars, the planets, the moon, and your cosmic place of birth.

Accumulating energy is essential, but you must know how to hold on to it and sustain it as well. The pakuas are the collection points. Focus on them and use visualization of nature to activate the power. Program yourself to recognize and utilize the various powers of water or fire. You can feel the center of your being as it is charged. Do not lose sight of the various powers and organs. Connect everything, not forgetting the elements. When you are able to do this, you actually have achieved a wisdom that will help you and all those around you. This kind of peaceful but powerful energy is picked up by others. You are able to call on the chi ball and accept it in the spirit of love, light, peace, and gratitude.

In the practice of Fusion, there is a strong emotional component. When the forces come together in the pakuas, all emotional negativity is neutralized. Negativity in the organs is transformed, becoming more refined and balanced. Consequently, it is stronger and more usable. One thing it is used for is to attract more Primordial Force. This is likened to becoming one with God, which can be thought of as transcendence.

Negative emotions can cause sickness. The source of emotions can be internal, external, or cosmic. Your total environment has an impact on your total being. When negativity is widespread it creates a society that is profoundly negative. It creates hatred, causes death, and even causes war. Much of the modern world suffers from this. Living a life where you emit negativity results in the accumulation of negativity; the price for this is quite high. But creating a positive force in society results in the opposite, which is goodness, health, happiness, and joy. There is a negative and positive component in all things, and the purpose in life is to balance by connecting with the Tao.

The way to bring about a peaceful and harmonious environment in practice is to connect daily to the forces of Mother Earth, connect with the heavenly force, establish a connection to the North Star, and download the violet light. Symbols, visualization, and mental constructs are the tools in your personal toolbox. You need to choose the one that works best for you and the situation you face. The one constant that you will find is the need to recognize and make good connections. You need to learn true gratitude so you can release your attention and give it over to a Higher Power. Release entails having trust and faith. It allows interaction because the proper connection has been established. You are then able to shield yourself from your anger and other negative emotions, so that suffering is gone and negativity recycled. Instead of destroying yourself, you are cultivating your vital force.

You were born with a mountain on your head, and you can visualize it with the antenna that allows you to request or download from the Prime Mover of the cosmos. You want to receive wisdom and knowledge because this is what educates the spirit and soul. As you connect to the violet light, energy can then begin to flow down like water into your organs (see fig. 2.34). This begins a cleansing process that removes all the negative thoughts and actions from you. Courage and righteousness result. You experience true gentleness and real peace.

Such powerful loving forces mean you are now capable of healing anything. You become a kinder and more generous person because positive forces are feeding your spirit and your soul. You have more courage and honor, thus you radiate peace, love, and understanding. The result is that chi grows all these positive forces. You must truly listen as you turn your senses inward in order to experience cosmic bliss. Everything is interconnected; doing these Taoist practices will

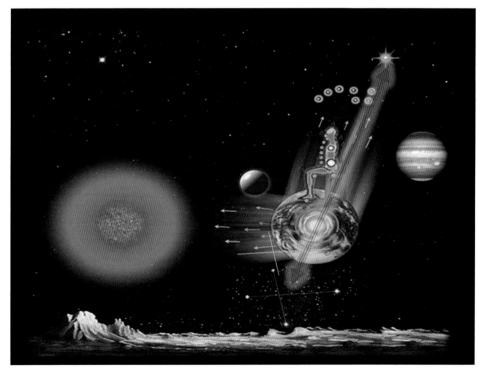

Fig. 2.34. Utilizing connections internally, you are able to connect to the violet light.

program your inner self to have the ability to activate all the connections with a simple act of will.

Doing all the internal work will expand your spirit and soul. The result is consolidation, stabilization, and enhancement as you become more balanced and in alignment with the Tao. The Fusion practice particularly serves to enhance maturity and positive energy in your organs and glands. Consequently the energy is pure and more usable for creating a positive environment. It is actually concentrated and is a form of compassion energy, formed as a pearl. When all types of positive energy come together as the fire of love and compassion, sexual energy is steamed and transformed into creative and spiritual energy. As a higher form of energy, this serves to nourish your physical body.

TAOIST ESOTERICS

You can see that there are two forms of energy. They can be viewed as physical energy and spiritual energy. While they emerged as two sides of the same coin, making a distinction between them makes it easier to grasp the wisdom of the Tao. Philosophers and scientists alike are well aware of the intimate connection between the mind and the body. Advanced forms of the Tao sometimes even talk about the spirit-body.

That is why looking inward and connecting outward is so critical. If you do your personal esoteric work correctly your position in the cosmic realm will be elevated. You acquire respect in the spiritual arena of your life. The overall position that you hold in this universe at this moment in time is simply that of a child. At the same time, the more highly developed in the esoteric methods of the Tao you are, the more honor and respect you get and the more you mature. The spirits and beings that are present in the cosmos help protect and educate you in terms of esoteric knowledge. It is then your responsibility to put this knowledge to use and gain experience.

Taoism is an extremely esoteric approach to many aspects of the spiritual and physical world. It has been evolving for thousands of years and has a history that is interwoven with diverse methods of meditation, medicine, and alchemy. It is a philosophy that emphasizes transcendence and connections with nature, other beings, and ultimate reality itself. The result is a lifting up of your being with better internal and transpersonal communication. You achieve a happier and healthier life based on expansion of the consciousness of external and internal reality.

Taoism approaches everything in a threefold fashion: the human, the earthly, and the cosmic. There is a rich assortment of symbolism such that the end result is total consolidation of the spirit, mind, and body, woven into a fabric rich in wisdom. Inner awareness utilizes both visualization and association, not just of the organs themselves, but also of the natural world. As you understand more and become wiser, each time you do these Taoist practices everything will become clearer and easier. Activation will be as simple as pushing a button. You will grasp the importance of the sexual practices of the Taoist masters. Upon remembering, activating, and visualizing the main bodily points of orgasmic power, you will heal yourself and make yourself less vulnerable to negativity both mentally and physically. You will create a positive aura that surrounds you and assists you in interacting with others.

It needs to be pointed out that enlightenment is not a once and for all proposition. It is not static. It is a journey, and there are stages of enlightenment. The practice of the Tao can be viewed as technical knowhow, and this is the first step of a million. Knowhow entails always enhancing your goal. The simple key is to understand that the point is to produce energy. Keep in mind that energy production is the result of sexual arousal. As with all energy, you must be charged in order to be able to function.

The Way of the Tao is cyclical in nature, as you can clearly see in the yin and yang symbol. Taoism is such a natural, scientific, and spiritual point of view that its fundamentals can be found in the teachings of all the great religions. That includes the Judeo-Christian perspective, which most in the Western world are quite familiar with. While the Bible lacks any discussion of specific practices, nevertheless it is possible to see a similar framework there. In particular there are many parallels between the teachings found in the New Testament and those found in the teachings of the ancient Taoist sages. Some have even postulated that Jesus travelled to ancient China and learned those teachings. Be that as it may, it is quite clear that all the great teachers throughout history have a great deal in common.

The point here, once again, is that the search for love, joy, and happiness allows for many viewpoints. The Bible says that God is love and this is in perfect accord not only with the practice of the Tao but with the teachings of everything from Buddhism to Islam. Being a wise person not only means that you choose what is wise but that you know what not to choose. Taoism, rather than threatening nonbelievers with hell, simply points out the polarity and balance of the cosmos. If your belief system facilitates love, joy, and happiness, then it is true. If your belief system facilitates fear, anxiety, guilt, and shame, then it is not correct because it forces you to live in a negative atmosphere that is out of balance.

Accessing the sexual power and using it to increase energy is something that has both personal testimonials as well as scientific corroboration to substantiate it. Unfortunately the energy that is produced utilizing orgasmic methods is something that is prohibited by some belief systems. Those who pursue the Taoist system need only remember that sex is natural and normal for all living beings. There is nothing shameful or evil about it. Once a personal awakening takes place, the practitioner can access this infinite source of chi.

Taoist sexual practices are utilized to rejuvenate and refresh the physical body as well as the spirit and soul. These practices will make you healthier and more youthful. The idea is this: sperm and eggs are essentially seeds that control hormones and blood. They can be utilized to manage personal energy. The Taoist system prevents energy from

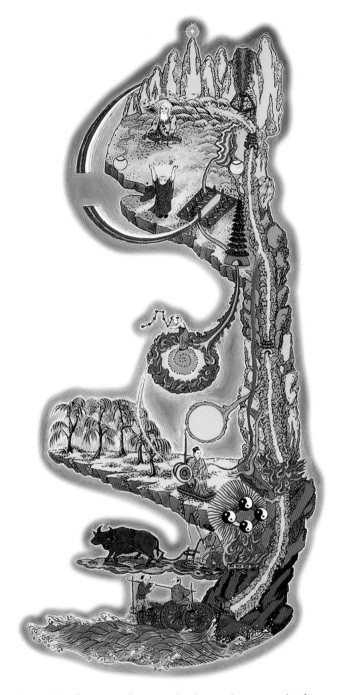

Fig. 2.35. The natural waterwheel (see the appendix for a
detailed explanation of this image)

being wasted. The cyclical nature is cause and effect. This is a natural waterwheel (see fig. 2.35). Inner Alchemy is the backdrop for the energy and transformative powers of the Tao. The energy is circulated in a more efficient fashion. Having opened the resources provided by the practice, you then create a personal aura exuding love, joy, and happiness.

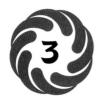

The Universal Healing Tao System

The evolution of the Universal Healing Tao system started innocently enough when a small high school boy in Hong Kong, China, encountered a Taoist mountain sage who had recently come down from the Himalayas in northern China.

I (Master Chia) first learned of the practices of Inner Alchemy (changing one substance into another) more than fifty-five years ago when I was in my first year of high school. My school friends and I enjoyed reading kung fu comic books and idolized the comic book characters. We were all fascinated and aspired to be like our comic book heroes with their incredible skills. Then one day we heard about a great Taoist sage who had arrived in Hong Kong. This Taoist sage, White Cloud (Yi Eng), had been forced down from the mountains because of the Chinese Counter-Cultural Revolution. The Chinese army was literally bombing many of the Himalayan mountain areas where Buddhist monasteries and Taoist temples had been built into the mountains for training and higher level practices. Several thousand monasteries were destroyed and millions of Buddhist monks and Taoist sages were killed during this period.

White Cloud had been living in the mountains in a cave for thirty years. He had gone there after studying in a northern Taoist temple. He had left the temple, seeking instruction in high-level practices, which he could not obtain there. He had been advised by his headmaster to seek a mountain sage to complete his training to be an Immortal. For his first six years in the Himalayan Mountains he wandered around looking for a sage to teach him. He nearly starved to death, as there is no food at that altitude in the mountains.

Finally he stumbled into a cave and saw a sage in a sitting meditation posture; he was not moving or visibly breathing. White Cloud could not believe his eyes. He prostrated himself, prayed, and showed praise continuously for weeks and months but nothing happened, as the sitting sage did not move. At last, the meditative sage, who had been out of his body, opened his eyes. But then he closed his eyes after seeing White Cloud and left again. White Cloud went crazy and prostrated himself, prayed, and showed praise continuously again. Weeks went by and White Cloud was beside himself with nowhere to go and no funds to get there. After another month or so the meditative sage opened his eyes again. Seeing White Cloud still there, he decided out of pity to teach him the Inner Alchemy system of practices.

Many years later, when the mountain refuges were being bombed, White Cloud went south to Hong Kong, a British colony at the time, seeking a peaceful place to resume his practices. My friends and I planned to go across town together to meet the Taoist sage on a given Tuesday to find out if he could teach us kung fu like in our comic books. But when that Tuesday arrived I was the only one who went. I knocked on the door. The door opened and the sage appeared. He looked at me and said, "I am going to teach you the Tao." So for the next four years, two to three days a week the Taoist sage taught me all of the Internal Alchemy formulas, refined from the amazing experiences of many generations of masters into nine practical stages of Taoist internal spiritual cultivation. Forty years later, I established the core practices of the Universal Healing Tao system from the original

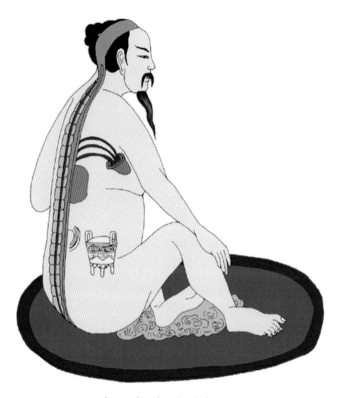

Fig. 3.1. Taoist Master White Cloud, who left his body at age ninety-six

Nine Inner Alchemy Levels given to me by Yi Eng (see fig. 3.1).

At the end of my senior year of high school, before I returned to my home in Bangkok, Thailand, I said goodbye to my Taoist master. White Cloud smiled and told me that one day I would move to the United States and start teaching the Tao and its Way. He made me promise that I would first teach the Tao to the Chinese in the U.S. for three years before beginning to teach it to Westerners. Nearly twenty years later, in 1976, I moved to New York City. I fulfilled my promise and taught Chinese students for three years, then began teaching Westerners. Highly refined states of inner experience and consciousness are the birthright of all humans and are accessible by all.

In my lineage, we call ourselves the "Inner-Alchemy-Just-Practice Taoists." People in this lineage take out what is not necessary, including all rituals and ceremonies. When White Cloud met my grandmaster, the master gave no initiation, no celebration, nothing at all—just pure practice. They combine all the things that are effective, usually learning from many systems, such as Hinduism, Buddhism, Islam, Christianity, and the science of today's world. Inner-Alchemy-Just-Practice Taoists go to the mountains, practice, and come down to teach and help people.

ORIGINAL NINE INNER ALCHEMY LEVELS OF TAOIST MASTER YI ENG (WHITE CLOUD)

The nine Taoist Inner Alchemy levels of immortality (丹九公式) are the core practices of the Universal Healing Tao system. They are the following: Primordial Force Activation, Sexual Alchemy, Fusion Alchemy, Lesser Kan and Li, Greater Kan and Li, Greatest Kan and Li, Sealing of the Five Senses, Congress of Heaven and Earth, and Reunion of Heaven and Man.

Our practice can lead to fruition only through a correct way of understanding. This means that we must view these nine levels together as the way, and understand how they connect to the Way of the Tao itself. *Tao* means "way": the way of nature and the universe, the natural way. The Way of the Tao is a process of returning to Wu Chi, the primordial all-conscious void. In this process the practitioner consciously senses the personal chi within the body, and then the chi of Earth, nature, and the universe. To understand the supreme Inner Alchemy of the union of human and Tao means to know the Way. To know the Way, one needs to know the positions of Heaven and Earth, like a man who goes out to hike in the forest uses a compass and a map. To perform the Inner Alchemy, we likewise need an inner map of our inner time and space, and an inner compass. We must know about the internal centers, organs, channels, and hormonal glands; that is, we must know the inner landscape and energy points. This knowledge is called inner feng shui: the inner maps are provided, step by step, in each of the levels. Going through each of these, one gets ready to understand the feng shui of the inner brain and the alchemy of developing the inner compass.

The first level provides the inner feng shui of the body's north-south axis and the Heaven and Earth polarity, the yin and yang flowing in their natural directions. Each consecutive formula of White Cloud's supreme alchemy introduces a more complete map of the inner body. When the knowledge of the inner feng shui, learned in the practice of Internal Alchemy, is applied to so-called external practices, like Chi Kung, those practices also become Inner Alchemy.

In Chinese, *Inner Alchemy* is called Nei Tan Kung (內丹工), which spells "internal elixir skill," meaning Inner Alchemy practice, and as such is contrasted with Wei Tan Kung or "external elixir skill." The term *External Alchemy* (Wei Tan Kung) is normally used for material or physical things, like Chinese medicine, Chi Kung exercise, and martial arts, but each of these can become internal as well, if the wisdom gained from the inner alchemical work is applied to the outer alchemical work. In the higher formulas, the distinction between internal and external is replaced by a multidimensional view, where different levels can be experienced at the same time. The boundaries of inner and outer are transcended once we enter the realm of Spiritual Alchemy, Nei Tan Shu (內丹術).

Some may find it interesting to hear that spiritual development can go hand in hand with a loving, respectful sexual relationship as well as solo cultivation practice. And further, that the sexual energy generated in the process is a critical element for spiritual development. One learns to cultivate, control, conserve, refine, and store sexual energy in the body in the first two levels: Primordial Force Activation and Sexual Alchemy. From there, the more refined Inner Alchemy practices enable Universal Tao practitioners to grow and attain their immortal spirit body. It begins with the Fusion energy (soul) body practices. Through Inner Alchemy processes, one refines the immaterial (sexual energy essence and healthy positive energy) generated from the material (physical body) and sources of Earth, nature, planets, and the universe. A practitioner can become energetically "pregnant." By intention one can create and nurture a crystalized energy "fetus" (using the physical analogy).

With loving attention and care from the upper hierarchy of meditation practices—Lesser, Greater, and Greatest Kan and Li, and Sealing of the Five Senses—one feeds, transfers consciousness, and trains this energy body to grow like a healthy child. The goal is to have time to accomplish the energetic refinement and crystallization of one's true spiritual self, referred to as the "golden light body" (golden is a reference to the high value accorded to this attainment, not necessarily its permanent color) (see fig. 3.2). It does not happen by whim or chance. It takes

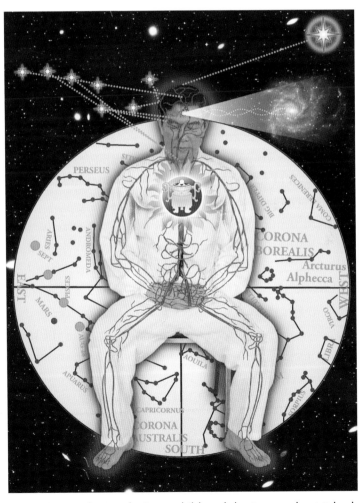

Fig. 3.2. Developing the inner child and the immortal spirit body

time, patience, and commitment. Therefore, Taoists value a healthy, happy, emotionally balanced life and longevity to support feeling good and being willing to persevere with this higher Inner Alchemy process.

The process is further refined in the practices of the Congress of Heaven and Earth and then the Reunion of Heaven and Man. The golden light body is one's immortal vehicle for spiritual freedom and independence. It transcends the limits of the physical world of time and space, even while one is still living in the here and now. The goal can be attained and experienced in this lifetime. It is the ultimate meaning and purpose of life!

First Inner Alchemy Level: Primordial Force Activation

White Cloud's First Formula of Inner Alchemy involves the Three Treasures: Heaven, Human, and Earth (天 Tian, Heaven; 人 Ren, Human; 地 Di, Earth) and their cosmic relationship. It teaches practitioners the first level of the inner feng shui: the Inner Smile, Microcosmic Orbit, Chi Self-Massage, and Six Healing Sounds.

The Microcosmic Orbit is an Inner Alchemy practice in which practitioners learn to circulate their chi, or life force, along the meridians of the front and back sides of the body known as the Governor and Conception Vessels. This first level is as simple as it is supreme, teaching us to become aware of Earth beneath our feet and Heaven above our crown, and to place the tip of our tongue on the roof of the palate, to connect the major yang and yin vessels of the body. Then we relax our mind and focus our attention downward into the body. As our mind relaxes, the chi or bioelectric energy can flow down from the head (yang = red) to connect into the Conception or Yin Vessel at the tip of the tongue (yin = blue). After some practice the flowing down of the chi can be clearly felt in the forehead and tasted on the tongue, first a tingling sensation like touching a battery. This is followed by the distinctly sweet tasting saliva, the inner alchemical nectar, which is produced as the chi flows down from the pineal gland into the Yin Vessel, activating all the glands of the endocrine system.

The Microcosmic Orbit continues to flow down from the throat center to the heart, solar plexus, navel, and sexual center. From the perineum, it connects to the Governor or Yang Vessel at the tail and sacrum bones, flowing along the spine back up to the crown, completing one round of the Microcosmic Orbit. The perineum also connects to the soles of the feet through the leg channels, completing the earth route. The earth force enters the leg channels at the beginning of the Kidney meridian, in a point (KD 1) at the center of the sole of the foot, called "Bubbling Springs" (see fig. 3.3).

The formula of the Microcosmic Orbit teaches us about the union of Heaven and Earth, and their relation to the Human, who physically, mentally, and spiritually has been born from the

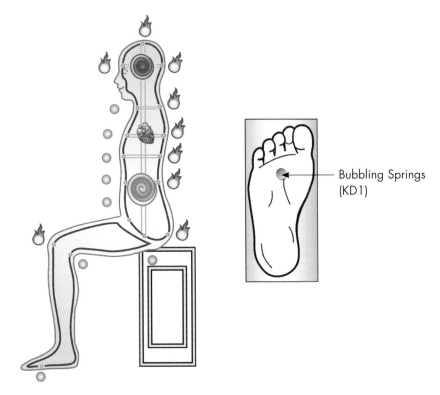

Fig. 3.3. Microcosmic Orbit and Kidney 1 point

alchemical marriage of Father Heaven and Mother Earth. The human body is a microcosmic reflection of the macrocosmos, as can be seen from the upright stature of the human being: the crown

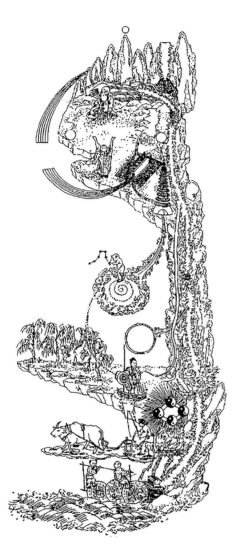

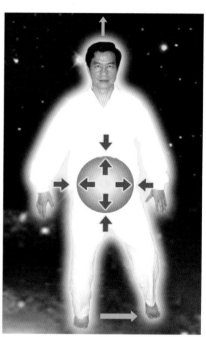

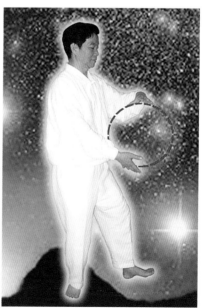

Fig. 3.4. The "small heavenly cycle" of the Microcosmic Orbit reflects the "great heavenly cycle."

of the head connects to Heaven, and the feet connect to Earth.

In Taoism it is said that "what comes down to Earth has to go up to Heaven, and what comes up to Heaven has to go back to Earth." In the human body, this "great heavenly cycle" is reflected in the "small heavenly cycle," or Microcosmic Orbit (see fig. 3.4). The way up to Heaven (the mountain) naturally corresponds with the spine, and the back side of the head, and the way down to Earth (the valley) corresponds with the front side of the body. The back side of the body is hard (yang) and the front side is soft (yin). It is natural for the yang to flow up and for the yin to flow down, hence the yin gathered to create Earth and the yang to create Heaven.

The inner feng shui of this formula focuses on the Governor and Conception Vessels and the stations, or points, along the vessels through which the Microcosmic Orbit travels. It also teaches how to connect through the crown with the Source, following the lead light to the North Star and the Big Dipper and beyond into the birth of the universe from the Wu Chi. This formula thus already prepares the student for the spiritual practices of the next formulas. Auxiliary practices like the Inner Smile, Chi Self-Massage, and the Six Healing Sounds are taught as part of the first level, because they help the chi to orbit and they help refine and cultivate our inner elixir, our Nei Tan (內丹).

The inner alchemical microcosmos (of the body), in relation to the outer alchemical macrocosmos, defines the placement and axis of the body, the Heaven and Earth poles, the north and the south. As soon as we start to move the body, the axis slides and thus east, west, and the intermediate corners come into play. With these eight directions and the zenith and the nadir (the up and down), there are ten macrocosmic dimensions to which the microcosmos of the body relates. Being in movement, the body exchanges energy with the forces of the ten directions. Through harmonizing the body's movements with this natural flow of energy (chi), the practice of Tai Chi Chi Kung is born.

Our microcosmic relationship with the earth is such that what we bring to the earth must bounce back to us. Through the internal practice of Chi Kung postures, it is possible to raise our awareness to the chi particles as they are bubbling up from the earth. Such practices are taught along with the first level, as the Microcosmic Orbit is applied to Chi Kung practice, and students first learn to circulate and store the energy in their own body (Iron Shirt Chi Kung) and later to absorb energy from outside and to discharge energy. The purpose of the external Chi Kung is to provide longevity: a sufficient length of time to attain the Internal Alchemy. The intention of Chi Kung is not to defend yourself but to support and activate inner transformation. The Taoist walks slowly and carries a big stick, which is the Chi Kung practices.

Second Inner Alchemy Level: Sexual Alchemy

The second level teaches the inner feng shui of the three tan tiens and the supreme Inner Alchemy of the Three Pure Ones (heavenly force, earth force, cosmic force). In Taoist tradition, it is said that the Three Pure Ones present the return to the Tao directly after the split of the Wu Chi into yin and yang. The cosmic force makes yin and yang stick together, and permeates the universe as the presence of cosmic love. In the microcosmic world of the human body, the Three Pure Ones manifest as the three tan tiens or the three Elixir Fields, and the inner alchemical process of the transformation of sexual energy, ching (精), into life force, chi (氣), and life force into spirit, shen (神). As such, Sexual Alchemy is about the transformation of the material into energy, and energy into spirit, but also about the transformation of spirit into energy and matter, hence procreation, the creation of bodies (see fig. 3.5). The conception of a human being is like the coming together of the three forces.

When our parents come to unite in love, the yin and yang orgasmic energies cross over and the cosmic force manifests as universal love, initiating the way of return to the Tao. At that moment, creation is repeated and the Heaven and Earth forces are drawn together, mixing with the hereditary Prenatal Chi of the ancestors, which is transmitted through the parents. This whirling spiral of cosmic forces uniting

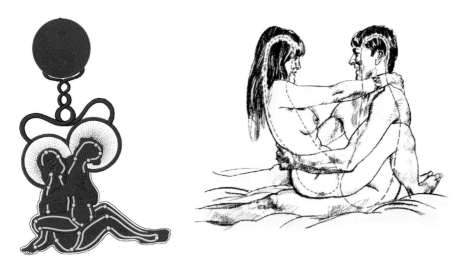

Fig. 3.5. Sexual Alchemy

is called the Primordial Force. From the moment of conception on, we continue to draw in chi from external sources, from the three forces and the food we receive from nature. At birth, we start to breathe the "Later Heavenly Breath" as we take in energy from the cosmic elements. After birth, when the umbilical cord is cut, the Prenatal Chi is stored with the Primordial Force in the lower tan tien, between the navel, sexual center, and kidneys. It is called the Original Chi because, once we are born, we cannot replenish this energy, and as we mature, we start to lose more and more of it. Our Original Chi, or our essence, ching, starts to leak out first at the onset of puberty, through menstruation and childbirth in women, and ejaculation in men. Later, factors of aging, unhealthy lifestyles, and stress can further diminish our Original Chi.

We can do nothing about this leakage of life force unless we know how to practice Sexual Alchemy. This divides into the practices of Single Cultivation, female and male, which unite in the supreme accomplishment, Dual Cultivation. Men learn to "Tame the White Stallion," to control the loss of life force through (unnecessary) ejaculation and to transform the sexual energy (ching) into life force (chi) and then transform it into spirit (shen). Women practice to "Slay the Red Dragon," to control menstruation, transform the blood into milk and milk into chi, and likewise transform it into spirit.

Through practices such as Testicle Breathing and Ovarian Breathing, Power Lock, and Orgasmic Upward Draw, students are taught to draw up the ching, the elixir, into the Microcosmic Orbit. Each station of the orbit refines and transforms the elixir, and thus the transformation into life force and spirit is realized. The Sexual Alchemy practice, performed on the path of Supreme Inner Alchemy, is in fact a spiritual practice as well as a "physical" practice, since it activates and regenerates the original force, yielding the elixir of physical immortality, and at the same time prepares the Immortal Fetus for the spiritual practice. The elixir of physical immortality is further cultivated in physical practices like Chi Kung and Tai Chi. The Immortal Fetus is nurtured and developed in the following level of White Cloud's Supreme Inner Alchemy.

Third Inner Alchemy Level: Fusion Alchemy

The third level of Inner Alchemy teaches the inner feng shui of the five elements and the eight forces. The dynamics of the five elements connect the microcosmos of the body with the elements, energies, and directions of the macrocosmos. This formula teaches how to establish a cauldron and form the pakua, as well as how to transform negative emotional qualities into neutral energy, by fusing the five elemental essences of the organs together. Elements that would otherwise clash on grounds of their "opposite" dynamics are fused in the inner alchemical cauldron, to yield the "superelement," the virtuous elixir called the pearl. The five elemental essences are drawn from the organs into collection points, and then spiraled into the spinning centers of the six pakuas, four on each side of the cauldron in the torso, one above, and one below. These energies mix with and are transformed and protected by the elemental forces of nature, the planets, and the eight primordial forces. The five elemental essences are transformed into a pearl, from which are produced virgin children (virtue energies) and protective animals.

In the practices of Cosmic Fusion and Fusion of the Eight Psychic Channels, the inner feng shui of the Central Channel, the two Thrusting Channels, the Belt Channels, and the Psychic Channels are taught (see fig. 3.6). Then the inner alchemical practice of circulating the pearl through the channels is introduced. The Central Channel runs from the crown to the perineum and passes right through the center of the cauldron, which for this formula is established at the navel center. The two Thrusting Channels run parallel to the Central Channel, on a line from the eye to the testicle or the ovary, both right and left. The Central Channel and Thrusting Channels can be used to quickly transport energy from the perineum to the crown and vice versa, and they are used in the higher formulas of the Kan and Li, to move the cauldron to the higher centers. The Belt Channels run all around the body and offer psychic protection together with the eight psychic channels, called the Bridge and Regulator Channels. Once the channels have been prepared, a special pearl is produced in the cauldron, which can be brought through the Central Channel into the crown, from where it is projected "out" to form the soul and spirit body. This pearl contains the seed for our Immortal Fetus, which must be impregnated with essential

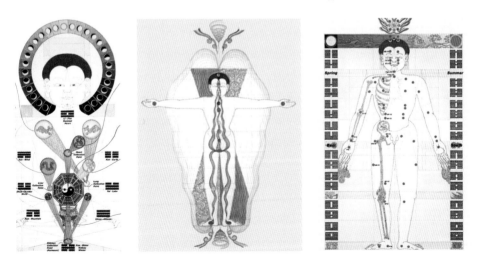

Fig. 3.6. Fusion of the Five Elements, Cosmic Fusion,
Fusion of Eight Psychic Channels

chi from the liver to yield the soul body. These practices are continued in the next three formulas, which entail transmutations of Kan (water) and Li (fire), taking place in the cauldron at different locations in the body and with ever-higher intensity.

Fourth Inner Alchemy Level: Lesser Enlightenment of Kan and Li

This level teaches the inner feng shui of reversing the positions of the fire and water elements in the body, the alchemical marriage and cooking of the elixir, and the steaming of the channels.

Lesser Enlightenment of Kan and Li, in fact an inner Sexual Alchemy practice, deepens the process of reunion with the Primordial Force. It nourishes, raises, and develops the Immortal Fetus, after its alchemical conception in Sexual Alchemy and Fusion Alchemy has taken place. The heart stores part of the Primordial Force. When these two combine together, they will form a more complete force. This process establishes a powerful "steaming" effect in the cauldron at the level of the navel center. This steaming is used to cleanse, purify, and strengthen the organs and brain to better attract the Primordial Force. Our Immortal Fetus is established in the tan tien. The elixir of immortality is prepared by reversing the usual sites of the water and fire element in the body: normally the fire in the body is up and the water is down. Following their natural course, the fire will flare up and the water will leak out and dry up. By placing the fire under the water and cooking the elixir, this formula actually teaches us the secret of the fountain of youth.

Fifth Inner Alchemy Level: Greater Enlightenment of Kan and Li

This level teaches the inner feng shui of drawing energy from macrocosmic sources: sun, moon, and planets. This is a further reunion with the Primordial Force. Another cauldron is established at the solar plexus to draw on the yin and the yang forces of the sun, moon, and planets, and to intensify the steaming process, begun in the navel cauldron. Our Immortal Fetus is impregnated with Earth Chi from the spleen, and our spiritual embryo is formed. The steaming process purifies the organs and helps us achieve emptiness; it also softens and clears the Thrusting Channels for our embryo's passage to the heart. Since the forming of the soul and spirit bodies is part of this level, other immortal practices, such as self-intercourse, astral flight, domestic animals, virgin children, and the twelve channels, Gathering the Pill, and transferring the consciousness to the energy and spiritual body, are taught under this level.

Sixth Inner Alchemy Level: Greatest Enlightenment of Kan and Li

This level teaches the inner feng shui of establishing a cauldron at the heart center (middle tan tien); celestial, soul, and spirit alchemy. Again the reversal of the usual sites of water and fire, and the coupling of the fire with the water by placing it under the cauldron, will lead to a more intense cooking and steaming. The spiritual embryo is impregnated with the third essential alchemical ingredient, 神 shen, or spirit, which resides in the Crystal Palace, in the center of the brain, thus receiving the influx of our higher consciousness or spirit. If conditions are right, our inner child is born from the womb of our heart in an ocean of bliss. The soul body is yin, and the spirit body is yang. The soul body serves as an earth cable, absorbing the yang energy from the heavenly "wire" down into the body and the cauldron. It also absorbs yin energy from the earth, to balance the yang energy absorbed from the heavenly bodies and our spirit body. The celestial soul and spirit alchemy, belonging to this formula, is performed by manifesting the intention to connect to relevant heavenly bodies and attracting the cosmic primordial forces needed for our inner alchemical processes to the appropriate locations of our body. Thus the development of our energy (soul) and spirit body is furthered (see fig. 3.7).

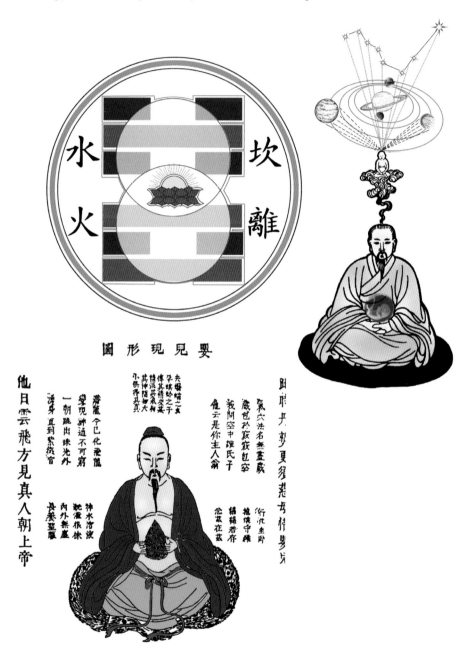

Fig. 3.7. Lesser, Greater, and Greatest Kan and Li

Seventh Inner Alchemy Level:
Sealing of the Five Senses

This level teaches the inner feng shui of establishing a cauldron at the mid-eyebrow point (upper tan tien), the inner alchemy of Sealing the Five Senses, and star and galaxy alchemy. The cauldron established at the mid-eyebrow point unifies the five shen, the five streams of personal consciousness that operate through our senses, with the five forces of the collective stellar self. The pure open space connecting the three tan tien cauldrons (at the navel, heart, and mid-eyebrow) is integrated. This stabilizes the celestial axis. Profound peace and different spiritual qualities continuously manifest from this activated core and radiate sonically into our physical being. Our senses are the openings of the spirit. If we constantly leak out and drain our spirit, depletion will drive our spirits out into the world, racing after new experiences and talking in the marketplace about what is rare to find, only to be left with more hunger. Emotions take up residence in our organs: anger occupies the mansion of the spirits, and frustrates the liver; hate settles in the heart, restricting the Hun Shen; anxiety about what may go wrong next eats at the spleen and starves the Yi Shen; sadness chases away the Po Shen and depresses the lungs; fear distills itself in the kidneys, drying out the Zhi Shen. Yuan Shen, our Original Spirit, has one last refuge: the brain. Given over to cunningness instead of truth, the heart then goes mad. As it says in the Tao Te Ching: "Five colors blind the eyes. Racing and hunting madden the heart. Pursuing what is rare makes action deceitful. The five flavors dull the palate, the five tones deafen the ears."

Eighth Inner Alchemy Level:
Congress of Heaven and Earth

This practice integrates the Early Heaven or formless self with the Later Heaven (Earth) physical self. Here the self identifies with two dimensions that coexist and co-create: the "formless form" of our being and the "substantial form" of our becoming. These two polar dimensions of our greater self engage in cosmic sex. They couple in order to reopen the portal to their original state, or "pre-self." This pre-state or Primordial Heaven is called Hundun, the primal chaos-unity that preceded the "Big Bang" of the cosmic egg cracking open.

The Three Treasures of Heaven, Earth, and Humanity are gathered in the three body cauldrons as Original Ching, Original Chi, and Original Shen. This three-tone harmonic chord is resonated with the fundamental or original tone of time and space. Consciousness then stabilizes in the axial center where our true multidimensional nature can now be embodied. This is symbolized by a tonal double vortex spinning faster than the speed of light within the void of space. Into this is fused our inner sage's immortal presence, the quintessence of humanity meditating in the center of a spiritual black hole. We must enter this portal to complete our journey of return to the origin.

Ninth Inner Alchemy Level: Reunion of Heaven and Man

This stage is the integration of the eight previous levels of consciousness into the experience of living simultaneously in the present moment in all dimensions, from physical linear time to spiritual eternal time. This state cannot be fully known or defined conceptually for others. Perhaps it might be conceptualized as the experience of living fully in the Wu Chi, the Supreme Unknown. It is the true achievement of the authentic or immortal self, a permanent state of grace known as Wu Wei, effortless action, or spontaneous action without acting. Creation (of the manifest) and return to formless origin seamlessly complete each other. Attainment of this ninth level is spontaneous, and happens when the inner will of our immortal sage within has reached complete alignment with the Tao. It usually occurs only by direct transmission from the Tao to the mature and receptive student, unless these Nine Inner Alchemy Levels are practiced together (see fig. 3.8).

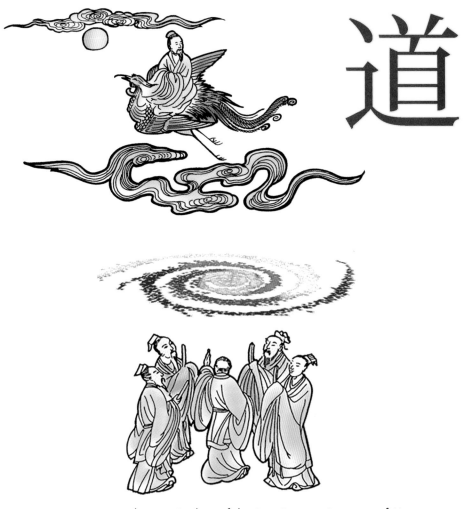

Fig. 3.8. Immortal Taoist Sealing of the Five Senses, Congress of Heaven and Earth, and Reunion of Heaven and Man

EXPANSION OF THE ORIGINAL NINE LEVELS

Using White Cloud's structure, I (Mantak Chia) have added my own refinements based on study with many masters as well as my studies in Western anatomy, astronomy, astrology, medical science, and the advancements in the field of quantum science, combined with my experience of over sixty years of practice and teaching.

To create a complete Internal Alchemy energetic system of practices, I added four levels of advanced Chi Kung practices—Iron Shirt Chi Kung, Tendon Nei Kung, Bone Marrow Nei Kung, and Tan Tien Chi Kung—and three levels of Tai Chi Chi Kung practices—Tai Chi Chi Kung I (Yang Slow Short Form), Tai Chi Fa Jin (Yang Discharge Form), and Tai Chi Wu Style. These additions work to build a strong and powerful temple to practice in for longevity—100 to 150 years—the length of time needed to do the practices to achieve Taoist Immortality. Through my research I also added two additional healing arts: Chi Nei Tsang with five levels of hands-on internal massage and Cosmic Healing with two levels of cosmic Chi Kung distance healing to keep the physical body balanced and efficient for longevity.

As the UHT system slowly evolved over fifty years, I also added Sexual Reflexology, Cosmic Nutrition, Elixir Chi Kung, Cosmic Detox, Laughing Chi Kung, Tao Yin, Stem Cell Chi Kung, Cosmic Vision, Wisdom Chi Kung, World Link Meditation, Sun and Moon Meditations, Taoist Astrology (Cosmic Astrology, Inner Alchemy Astrology, and Five-Element Astrology), Taoist Philosophy (Living in the Tao, Secret Teachings of Tao Te Ching, and Taoist Shaman), again for longevity.

The Universal Healing Tao system is designed to cultivate a balanced life of love, health, longevity, and spiritual evolution (see

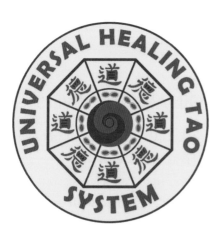

Fig. 3.9. The logo of the Universal Healing Tao system: the repeating Chinese characters in the logo mean "the Tao of Virtues."

fig. 3.9). It is a complete system for our integrated physical, energy (emotional), mental, and spiritual bodies. The focus is on developing and refining our life energy, chi (our bio-electromagnetic life force), for self-healing and life enhancement. We establish a relaxed, healthy base of life in our physical and social environment. At the same time, we strive to achieve spiritual independence and merge into oneness with the Wu Chi.

UHT Certification

To fortify and preserve the Universal Healing Tao system, the UHT Instructor and Practitioner Certification system was created and developed in the Four Healing Arts:

- **Living Tao** (Associate Instructor, Certificate Instructor, Senior Instructor)
- **Chi Nei Tsang** (Practitioner, Advanced Practitioner, Assistant Teacher, Teacher, Senior Teacher)
- **Cosmic Healing** (Practitioner, Advanced Practitioner, Assistant Teacher, Teacher, Senior Teacher)
- **Immortal Tao** (Inner Alchemy Instructor, Senior Instructor)

If you are looking for clarity, meaning, and purpose in life and would like to cultivate health, healing, happiness, and higher self-development , the Universal Healing Tao system provides a complete set of personalized tools to enable you to achieve your goals. You will also be aided to transform the frustrations of stress and tension into vitality for a full life, and to access reality-based experiences of the spiritual dimensions within. Whether a complete novice or an intermediate wandering truth-seeker, you already have the resources that you need to reach your goals. You just need to learn how to cultivate them, simply, step by step with the Universal Healing Tao system and its Taoist philosophy and astrology books, detailed in the bibliography.

UNIVERSAL HEALING TAO SYSTEM
FOUR HEALING ARTS CHART

LIVING TAO (EMOTIONAL BODY)

Basic Practices

- Inner Smile (Feel Internal Energy)

- Microcosmic Orbit (Functional and Governor Channels)

- Simple Chi Kung (Open Internal Energy)

- Six Healing Sounds (Cooling Internal Energy)

- Chi Self-Massage (Open Blockages)

- Cosmic Nutrition (Five-Element Nutrition)

Intermediate Practices

- Laughing Chi Kung (Open Heart Energy)

- Elixir Chi Kung (12 Postures) (Saliva—Water of Life)

- Activate Three Tan Tiens (Fires)

- Connect with Six Directions (Energy Fields)

- Tao Yin (Breath) (12 Yoga Posture Sets)

- Iron Shirt Chi Kung (6 Postures) (Alignment–Rooting–Packing)

- Tan Tien Chi Kung (12 Postures) (Dragon and Tiger Breath)

- Tai Chi Chi Kung (13 Movements) (Yang Slow Short Form)

- Stem Cell Chi Kung (Stem Cell Growth)

- Cosmic Vision (37 Eye Exercises)

Advanced Practices

- Tendon Nei Kung (8 Postures) (Tendon Growth)

- Bone Marrow Nei Kung (Growing Bone Density and Marrow)

- Tai Chi Fa Jin (15 Movements) (Yang Discharge Form)

- Tai Chi Wu Style (8 Directions) (Wu Style Tendon Growing)

Sexual Alchemy

- Male Sexual Management (Testicle Breathing)

- Multi-Orgasmic Man (Scrotal Compression)

- Prostate Chi Kung (Genital Massage, Orgasmic Upward Draw)

- Multi-Orgasmic Woman (Ovarian Breathing/Compression)

- Healing Love (Women) (Breast and Genital Massage)

- Jade Egg Exercise (Women) (Chi Weight Lifting)

- Uterus Chi Kung (Orgasmic Upward Draw and Power Lock)

- Multi-Orgasmic Couple (Dual Cultivation)

- Taoist Foreplay (Dual Cultivation)

- Sexual Reflexology (45 Healing Love Postures)

UNIVERSAL HEALING TAO SYSTEM
FOUR HEALING ARTS CHART (continued)

Fusion Alchemy

- Fusion of the Five Elements (Building Composting Machine and Pearl)

- Cosmic Fusion (Creative, Thrusting, and Belts Channels)

- Fusion of Eight Psychic Channels (Opening Bridge and Regulatory Channels, Spinal Cutting, Spinal Microcosmic Orbit, Aura Cutting, Crown Drilling, Aura Sealing)

- Advanced Fusions (Energy and Spirit Bodies Practices)

CHI NEI TSANG (PHYSICAL BODY)

Basic Practices

- Chi Nei Tsang (Open Up Energy Gates) (Internal Organ Massage)

- Cosmic Detox (Open and Cleanse Orifices)

Advanced Practices

- Advanced Chi Nei Tsang (Releasing Sick Winds)

- Chi Nei Ching (Spinal Massage and Tok Sen)

- Karsai Nei Tsang (Genital Massage)

- Life Pulse Massage (Restoring Blood Flow)

COSMIC HEALING (ENERGY BODY)

Basic Practices

- Cosmic Chi Kung (Hand Techniques)

- Cosmic Healing (Cosmic Energy)

Intermediate Practices

- Taoist Astral Healing

- Wisdom Chi Kung (Feed Brain with Cosmos)

- Cosmic Orbit (Macrocosmic Orbit with Cosmos)

- World Link Meditation (Linking to Other Practitioners)

- Sun Meditation (Violet/Red) (Cosmic Dust Particles)

- Moon Meditation (Silver/White) (Silver Saliva Elixir)

- Tree Chi Kung (Recycling Sickness Energy)

UNIVERSAL HEALING TAO SYSTEM
FOUR HEALING ARTS CHART (continued)

IMMORTAL TAO (SPIRITUAL BODY)

Basic Practices
(Fire and Water Practices)

- Lesser Kan and Li (Navel Cauldron)
- Darkness Technology (24/7 Darkness Practice)
- Greater Kan and Li (Solar Plexus Cauldron)
- Pi Gu Chi Kung (Energy Fasting)
- Greatest Kan and Li (Heart Cauldron)

Intermediate Practices

- Sealing of Five Senses (S5S) (Crystal Room Cauldron)

Advanced Practices
(Highest Inner Alchemy)

- Congress of Heaven and Earth
- Reunion of Heaven and Man

TAO GARDEN HEALTH SPA AND RESORT

Founded by Master Mantak Chia, the Tao Garden Health Spa and Resort is a worldwide center for Taoist training and holistic healing, detoxification, and rejuvenation. Located in the foothills of the Eastern Himalayas in the northern Thailand countryside near Chiang Mai, Tao Garden offers year-round Taoist training plus complementary health services. Both TCM (traditional Chinese medicine) and Ayurvedic modalities are integrated with limited Western medical services. Additionally, the Health Spa offers a full range of Thai massage, Ayurvedic massage, Chi Nei Tsang and Karsai massage, physiotherapy, hydrotherapy, and yoga. There is also a large swimming pool, gym, and other recreational facilities. Guests enjoy their time at Tao Garden in the beautiful surroundings of nature with fresh air, good water, and a delicious organic diet (see figs. 3.10 and 3.11). Our motto is: "good chi, good heart, good intention."

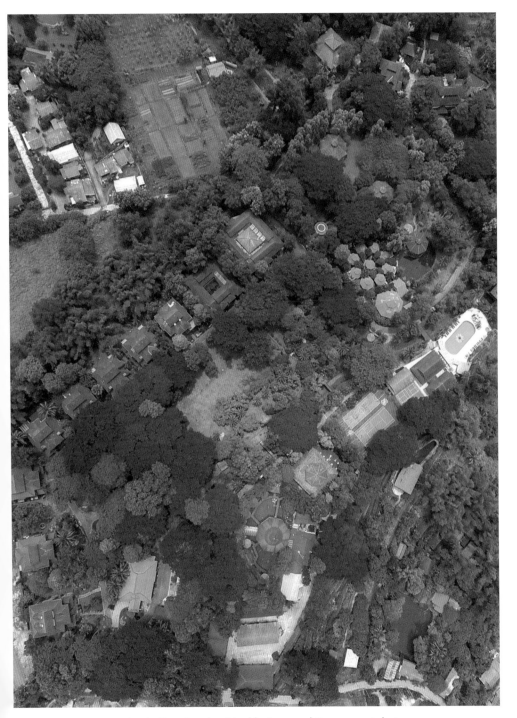

Fig. 3.10. Tao Garden Health Spa and Resort aerial view

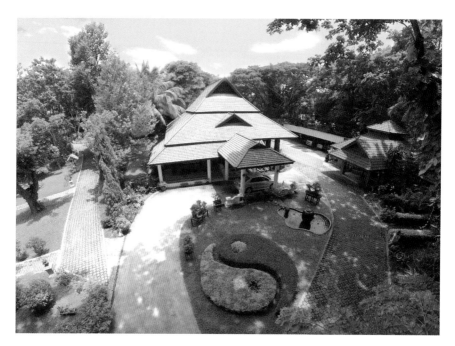

Fig. 3.11. Tao Garden Health Spa and Resort Reception

Master Chia teaches the Inner Alchemy levels during the summer and winter retreats held at Tao Garden every year (see figs. 3.12, 3.13, and 3.14). The higher Inner Alchemy formulas, which traditionally were practiced in caves, are taught in a complete darkness environment, which has been specially created to facilitate the teaching and practice of higher level Taoist alchemical meditation. These darkness retreats are only offered during the winter retreats, held annually in February.

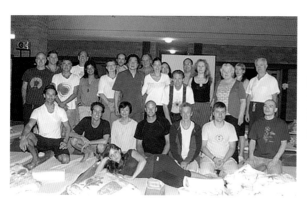

Fig. 3.12. A darkness retreat at Tao Garden before the lights are turned off

For a full overview of the summer and winter retreats, and more information about Tao Garden Health Spa and Resort, please visit www .tao-garden.com.

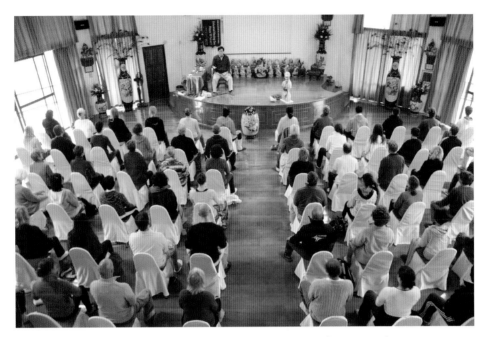

Fig. 3.13. Master Chia teaching Fusion meditation at the Immortal Meditation Hall at Tao Garden

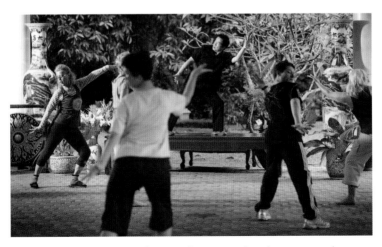

Fig. 3.14. Master Chia teaching Tai Chi Chi Kung at the Tai Chi Pavilion at Tao Garden

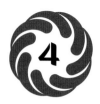

Primordial Force Activation

Taoist history goes back to the time when everybody was living in nature and in caves. They discovered what we call the Wu Chi, the Original Force or Primordial Force. In the Taoism of our lineage, the origin goes back to the Wu Chi, the supreme natural power in the universe—in Western terminology, God. It means "nothingness," but it is filled with dark matter, the subtle subatomic entities. Humans also store part of the Primordial Force. Starting from the beginning of conception when the egg and sperm come together, the first cell has the power to draw the Primordial Force down, combine with it, and form what comes to be a human. When the first cell divides and multiplies, the subsequent copies from the original retain the capacity to draw in the Primordial Force.

The whole Taoist practice is involved with how to evoke the Primordial Force in order to be reunited with it in our body. Primordial Force fills the whole universe. Dark matter is about 96 percent of the universe, and the other 4 percent is our physical universe. Each galaxy is a part of the Primordial Force, especially our galaxy, our solar system, and our planet Earth. Our solar system is just one out of 200 billion combinations of star and planet solar systems in our Milky Way galaxy. The Taoist understandings state that our Earth is the energy center of the galaxies of our universe. This point of view is supported by the most advanced science of today in the field of quantum mechanics. According to quantum theory, one quality of subatomic particles is "non-locality." With zero-point fluctuation as the underlying mechanism acting on quantum entities, causing one entity to affect the others, every part of the universe can be in touch with every other part instantaneously. These scientists believe that the "zero-point field" is the all-pervasive ground state throughout the universe. So it really doesn't matter where we are—we are at the center of the universe!

Thus, we are well-positioned and well-suited for the all-important process of drawing upon the Primordial Force for our life maintenance, refinement, and evolution. Fortifying ourselves with this essential resource enables us to manifest the amazing wonders of our human birthright. According to the Tao, the universe sends energy to Earth so Earth can support life. Earth stores a major part of the energy that we need in order to fulfill our birthright. Our planets also have a lot of influence on us, and all the planets store some of the elemental qualities of Primordial Force that we need to access in order to complete our inner alchemic transformation.

Most of the Primordial Force activation practices pertain to the emotional body and thus come under the "Living Tao" healing art. However, some Primordial Force activation practices affect the physical body and energy body, coming under the healing arts of "Chi Nei Tsang" and "Cosmic Healing," respectively. The Primordial Force activation practices that affect the emotional body are divided into basic, intermediate, and advanced practices. The Primordial Force activation practices for the physical body and energy body have similar categories.

LIVING TAO (EMOTIONAL BODY): BASIC PRACTICES

In order to activate the Primordial Force, we need to purify the organs and learn grounding to the earth. The basic practices that enable us to do so are: Inner Smile, Microcosmic Orbit, Chi Self-Massage, and Six Healing Sounds. Two other basic practices for Primordial Force activation are Simple Chi Kung, which is primarily breathing methods to open and energize the lower tan tien, and Cosmic Nutrition (Five-Element Nutrition).

Inner Smile

The Inner Smile is one of the most simple and powerful tools for healing. It uses the power of smiling to activate the relaxation response in the parasympathetic nervous system, thus fostering the disposal of negative emotions and rebalancing of positive emotions. When we learn to smile to the negative and make friends with it, we can find a way to live in harmony and enhance our health. Transforming negative emotional energy patterns into positive components in the organs helps to reprogram the genes and DNA.

You are a unique individual and your life experience is your own, so you need to search for and determine your own approach, utilizing the basic structure that is outlined here. Listen to your own heart and focus with your own mind. The Inner Smile is actually a form of inner communication, inner observation, and inner radiance. The world as we know it is very advanced in terms of communication, but for the most part inner communication is largely ignored. You also have your own form of inner communication with a vast network of nerves and blood vessels in the body, which can be developed.

Some people talk of the end times and the end of the world. The worst thing that is happening in today's world is that people do not understand the connections that they have in their own bodies, but they pay a lot of attention to their cell phones. The ancient Taoist texts tell us that you must look within yourself. At the time they were written there was little understanding of human anatomy, yet the Taoists were able to envision this science.

In the Inner Smile, the upper mind connects to every single organ. If you touch an organ, for example the liver, you can see it in your mind's eye and know the connection, not just to the brain but to the heart and other organs. Your inner eye looks at the liver and consequently you are in touch with the liver in a literal and a mental sense. The deeper you go into the body, the more you realize that it is full of energy (see fig. 4.1).

The organs are assigned different colors. These distinctions allow you to understand the emotional energy that is inside you. Western science is accepting the fact that emotions are not just in the brain but in all the organs. Love, for example, is everywhere inside you. Additionally

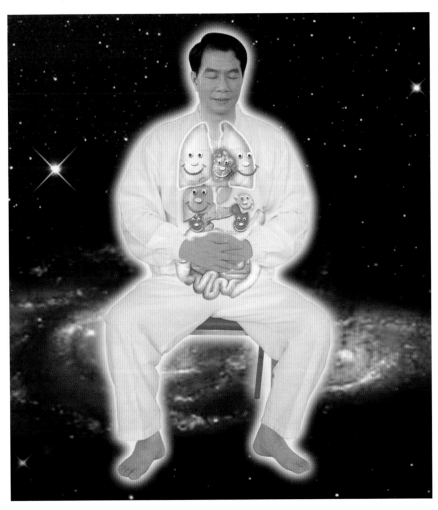

Fig. 4.1. Visualize your inner energy connecting with your vital organs.

joy and happiness are in you. Science says it is an actual fact that love is in the heart; it is not just poetry.

Much of the perspective of Western thought involves either blaming sin on the devil or, in a somewhat more sophisticated fashion, using psychology to say that a person has emotional problems because of bad parents or a bad environment. In the one case the solution is to claim that the devil needs to be banished and destroyed. In the other case, the recommendation is to wash or cleanse the mind. A close examination shows that neither of these things is realistic or possible. We know that suppressing emotions does not work either; in fact it causes sickness. Prisons and mental health facilities abound with little improvement of the overall problem.

Taoism does not utilize this framework of understanding. Instead, the Taoists understood that the negative and the positive coexist. Balance is the key. Negative cannot exist without positive and positive cannot exist without negative. You cannot have acid without alkaline. Scientists know that Earth must be balanced. You cannot make sense of the Tao without understanding this basic concept of balance.

The point of view of Taoism is that people need to take responsibility for their own condition and their emotional health. You and only you are responsible for your own life. You must choose the right path. In order to do this wisdom is required. If you do not approach things wisely you will get lost in the wilderness. You not only need to balance your organs but you need to balance your emotions, which are the expressions of your vital organs. Hatred, anger, jealousy, and other such emotions are negative and cause an imbalance. Smiling is one key, and it is possible for everyone. In addition to the outer smile, you have the Inner Smile. This smile helps you with your emotions and it puts you in touch with your organs. It enables you to get in touch with your internal body.

Your emotions come from the different organs, which store your long-term memories. Your brain is like a computer and the organs are the hard disks. The stress cycle starts with the liver. The emotions that are stored there are anger, envy, and jealousy, along with the associated stress. At the same time, courage, righteousness, and sincerity are stored there too, connecting with the lungs. If you are able to turn inward and smile to the liver, you can activate the positive forces in your body.

Suppression of negativity is particularly dangerous because the end result is an explosion. Again and again balance is the key. Your life is juggling balance. Wood produces fire, but what kind of fire it is depends on balance. It can be an angry and cruel fire or it can be a fire of love, joy, and happiness. Hatred is a profoundly negative emotion and it does not release quickly. It needs time. The heart is the storage place of love, joy, and happiness. You need to multiply your love so that you can share it. If everyone did that we would have a world of peace instead of war.

Wisdom starts with knowledge of yourself and your organs. Know yourself and you will be wise. You need to feel love, joy, and happiness, and if you do you will smile. The smile comes from within you. Those who go looking for gods or goddesses outside themselves will fail because God is in you. It is possible to eliminate anxiety and worry, but it is increasingly difficult in the modern world. One example of this stems from the realization that the earth contains metal and this is connected to your lungs. Your lungs have the potential to create depression. Because humans need images, knowing what your lungs look like is helpful. Know how they work and what they are related to. The body is your temple. Take care of it.

You also need to have knowledge of your kidneys. The negative emotions related to the kidneys include fear, shock, and trauma. There is a connection between the kidneys and the bones. Fear tries to squeeze your life force out. It makes you so cold that you shiver. The end result of fear is the loss of your Original Chi.

All of this relates to emotional wisdom, which stays with you for your entire life. There is only one person who can handle your emotional problems or imbalanced organs in the long run, and that is you. You are the one who has connections to the universe. We each have three universal gifts that are of great assistance in being emotionally wise:

1. The universal gift from the sky or the heavens
2. The universal gift of unconditional and unlimited love
3. The universal gift of the violet light

The universe has wisdom, unconditional and unlimited love, and finally it has the violet light. That is what you can get from the universe and you can consider that as a gift that is for you. You have the necessary connection in your being for self-discovery, but it is up to you to utilize it. What you request is of great importance. It is like the story of King Solomon. God asked Solomon what he wanted and all that Solomon requested was wisdom. King Solomon went on to become one of the richest kings in history. Everything comes from and is the result of wisdom.

The brain can receive wisdom and the heart can receive love. When you multiply love you need to begin with yourself. You need to do this to recognize and appreciate the highest light, which is the violet light. You can then love the people near you. First you love yourself, love your family and friends, and finally you can love your enemy. It is impossible to love your enemy without first loving yourself. Your heart was born with love, joy, and happiness and the ability to be connected to the Source. In addition it was born to be multiplied and finally to shine the radiant violet light.

You are limited as a person until you begin to make connections. The ultimate connection is to the unlimited source. Then you love and shine the violet light to others. In that way you eventually share your love with the universe. You can use the Inner Smile to share the love (see fig. 4.2). If you share the love, the love will return to you. What matters most is the energy, and it is possible for you to get this from others and even from the cosmos itself. Smile at the moon and you will get the energy of the moon. You will get nothing by shouting at the moon or the sun or the planets. You need to remember to be shining and radiant.

You begin the Inner Smile by holding your hands near your heart and smiling from your heart. Be very aware of your location both inwardly and cosmically. Smile to your heart. Within your body is wisdom, and you now know that your heart stores love, joy, and happiness. That is what everyone wants. Relax and smile again to your heart while

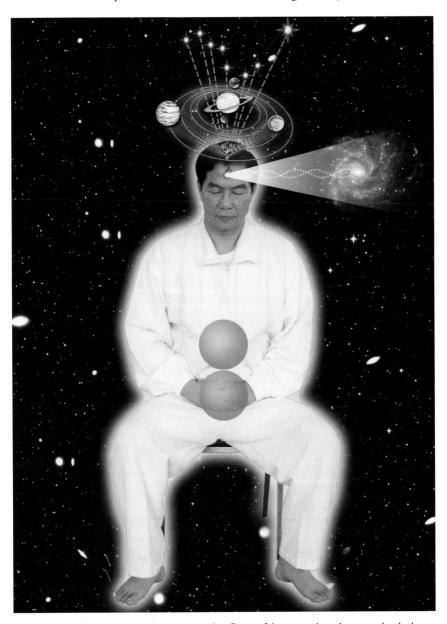

Fig. 4.2. The Inner Smile initiates the flow of love and radiant violet light.

inside your heart smiles to your Original Spirit. The radiance will begin to shine from you as you scan your environment. You are searching for the signal and your heart will recognize it. The heart is like an antenna; it stores your Original Spirit, which comes from above and the Supreme Creator. The Creator is right there inside you and shines the violet light and radiates the Inner Smile to individuals and creation.

Now you can get your blessing if you ask for the right thing. The right thing is wisdom. The light from the universe shines wisdom into your brain, then follows the path of your inner journey. You can then know that you have followed the right path. You feel the light in your small intestine; then it moves to the spleen and pancreas. You radiate openness and trust. The light then moves to your heart and lungs. It moves to your large intestine and courage is activated. Your kidneys and bladder are then activated and peace as well as silence is activated. You can then visualize your gallbladder and liver. You are now able to be virtuous and balance out the negativity. Finally you return to the heart and brain, and you have left anger behind you.

In the second stage you wrap the violet light about your spine and your saliva becomes energy-filled. You swallow so as not to lose the energy it contains. You continue to download love. Look at those you love—your family and your friends—and shine the love on them. As you activate your navel, you still have unlimited universal love. This becomes your entire way of being and your life's work. You always keep in mind that the key player with the Inner Smile is the heart, along with the universal Source: the provider of unconditional love. The renewed energy allows you to love yourself more, then others, and then the cosmos.

A close look at the liver will help to explain the effect of the Inner Smile on all the organs. Blockages of the liver can cause serious emotional disturbances, such as anger, frustration, and depression. The result of such negative emotions is reduced chi. The good news is that it is possible to change this energy back to positive life forces, bringing chi into your liver. Your organs do not work in isolation. Just like the cosmos itself, everything is connected. Your liver can fuel the fire in your heart. With lack of activity, negative thoughts, unhealthy food, or other factors, people sometime have a weakened connection to the Primordial Force, which causes an imbalance in the body. The solution for this is to do the Inner Smile. The negativity is recycled to Mother Earth and in return you get positive energy and refreshed chi, which enables you to manage the negative emotions. If your liver is hard you will experience difficulties, but you can soften it with your Inner Smile. Smile into your liver, which is located on the right side, just below your rib cage. Smile and fill it with your love. This restores chi and it helps facilitate health, happiness, and gifts to your life (see fig. 4.3).

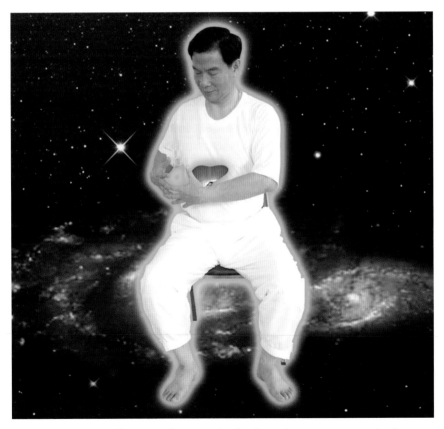

Fig. 4.3. Visualize your liver, and refresh and rejuvenate it with chi.

You follow the seasons. The heart is summer: shiny and radiant. The associated organ is the small intestine. Indian summer involves the spleen, stomach, and pancreas. Winter is next with the kidney and bladder. Spring follows that with the liver and gallbladder. That is the wisdom of the organs. Once the heart is involved you can move to any organ you choose, but the heart is required because of love. Without love you have no smile. The lungs are the beginning of the chi with the breath, which is needed for the smile too. Below is a step-by-step guide for the practice.

Simplified Inner Smile

1. Sit near the edge of your chair. Your feet should be flat and your back straight.
2. With your eyes, concentrate on the soles of your feet and their connection to the earth. Gently rock your spine.
3. Maintain a positive image in your mind. Activate your mid-eyebrow by massaging and pushing it, then relaxing and feeling it open.
4. See the smiling energy in front of and around you. Breathe it into your eyes.
5. Smile down to nose, cheeks, and mouth. Relax, gathering sweet and fragrant saliva in your mouth. Feel the smiling energy flow down your face as you relax. Feel it in your neck as you move your head side to side.
6. Smile to throat, thyroid, parathyroid, and thymus.
7. Smile to heart, radiating out love, joy, and happiness extended to the universe.
8. Feel joy and love spread to the lungs, liver, spleen, pancreas, kidneys, and genitals.
9. Smile down the whole body simultaneously, feeling the chi like a cooling waterfall of cosmic energy, smiles, joy, and love.
10. Smile to your navel as you cover it with your hands. Spiral with mind or hands 36 times outward (diaphragm to pubic bone), then inward back to navel 24 times.

You need not be in a hurry with this practice. Love your organs and feel them fill with chi. You will be filled with love, and all anger and frustration will be recycled to Mother Earth. Hatred, thoughts of cruelty, arrogance, and violence will dissipate. Everything will become smiling, loving energy.

☸ Special Focus on Lungs

Your lungs are a major part of the temple in your body. This exercise will help heal and keep your lungs healthy (see fig. 4.4).

1. Rock side to side and look left and right. Start by inhaling while raising the arms above the head. Hold your breath and visualize your lungs. At first they may seem cloudy and gray.
2. Smile inwardly and exhale. As you exhale release all negativity to Mother Earth. As you repeat this your lungs will grow clearer and whiter.

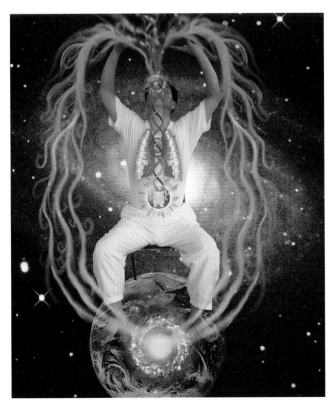

Fig. 4.4. Do lung exercises to keep your lungs healthy.

Microcosmic Orbit

Having a thorough understanding of the concept of orbits is key to Taoist practice. Such an understanding alone has the capability of resolving many issues and problems that people face in their daily lives. All things have orbits and are connected to each other. In terms of astronomy, we know about the orbits of the stars and planets. The moon orbits the earth and the earth orbits the sun. This has been consistently true for billions of years. The orbits are very predictable and our calendars are the result of the consistency of these orbits.

At the same time, there are orbits within you. You are made up of atoms and the atoms themselves have electrons that are spinning in orbit. Each cell contains more orbits than stars in the sky. If you connect the orbits within your body to external orbits, they influence the orbits within. This plays a significant role in the energy that you have within your being.

Remember, the only type of energy that can be utilized to replenish your being is sexual energy. The more chi you have the more chi you can make. This is a cornerstone of the practice. This is the cycle of chi and the fundamental orbit is the secret to life. Conserve, recycle, and transform. Sexual energy is key, but it needs to be cultivated, as it does not last long by itself. In the Microcosmic Orbit practice, sexual energy is multiplied by combining it with fire (heart–yang) and water (kidneys–yin). To do this we need to create a container or chi ball to hold the energies. As the four Tai Chi balls spin, they activate the yang and yin exchange, creating a chi ball.

As you circulate the chi ball in the Microcosmic Orbit, the energy spins and grows; therefore you have additional energy throughout your body. You simply sit on the coccyx, rock a little, hold your breath and then relax. Next you pull the sexual energy up to the brain. First it goes to the base of the skull and then to the crown. From there it drops down into the brain. You will experience the amazing power of sexual energy as it revitalizes your brain. You can tap your crown to assist the energy in flowing downward to complete its mission of revitalization. Next is the mid-eyebrow. Then you let the energy flow to your tongue and heart and through your body. The chi flow will energize your entire being as the four forces spin.

You repeat this process of circulating and spinning several times, guiding the chi to the appropriate organs in order to bring about rejuvenation. Following this you sit back in your chair and place your fingers on your navel. You will be recharging and healing yourself. When you focus like this you are opening blockages and the pain is released from your body. You are charging and healing at the same time. Opening the Microcosmic Orbit should be done at home to maintain some consistency in the cosmic treatment. There are three steps in opening up the Microcosmic Orbit:

1. Open the navel and the Door of Life.
2. Open the coccyx and the sacral pump.
3. Open the spine and connect to the cranium.

Once these have been accomplished, you can move to the other mechanisms: tapping, bringing the energy to the mid-eyebrow, opening the eyes, bringing the energy back down to the throat, heart, and navel again. This process can take several weeks or even months.

Preliminaries to the Microcosmic Orbit

Because your life has so many orbits there are many types and directions of spinning. Internally, you are generating chi. You can spin and orbit your own body simply by moving in a circular fashion. As you loosen your feel your sacrum and lumbar moving (see fig. 4.5 on page 146).

As you circle your body, be sure to move your eyes too. Eye movement is very significant in regard to the Microcosmic Orbit. There is a major connection between the eyes and the brain, and this connection is something that can be utilized in recognizing and amplifying the Microcosmic Orbit. You hold the chi ball in front of you in your mind

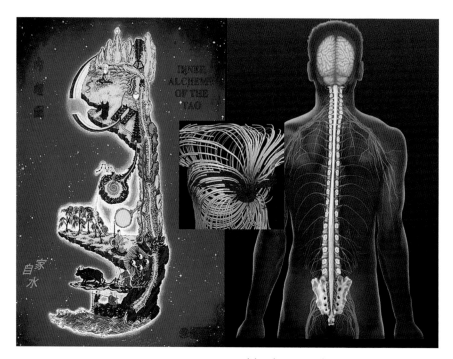

Fig. 4.5. Loosening your spine and lumbar vertebrae helps to connect you with your Primordial Force.

and circulate it, following it with your eyes. You simply need to truly focus on what you are doing. Notice that the term is *focus*; taken literally, that has to do with your eyes. You also have your mind that needs to be functioning properly in order to focus. The eyes are the director. They have the power. The energy you create has intelligence and it has the ability to repair your body.

All of your soldiers are in the form of white blood cells and all necessary healing aspects in your body are activated by being focused. The heart is also of great importance, but your army starts to march with the direction of your eyes. Every day you need to activate the eyes, mind, heart, spirit, and soul and then focus. This is how you develop consciousness. You then lower this down to the tan tien, which can be called the command post. You spin the chi ball forward and then spin it backward (see fig. 4.6). Mind, eye, and heart connect

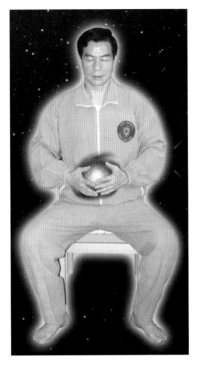

Fig. 4.6. Spin the chi ball at the tan tien.

at the mid-eyebrow. The heart is the commander, the liver is second in command, and the spleen is third. The lungs are fourth and the kidney fifth. The mind is like the prime minister and must be listened to as well, because on many matters it is the final authority. The eyes then commence to carry out the orders that have been given by the chain of command.

The faster the orbit goes, the more positive energy is created and the less negative energy is present. The orbit gets bigger and bigger. As you sit there the energy from the entire universe begins to affect you. There is a distinct pattern that is followed, and if you know this pattern you can understand it. Simply recognize that the pattern runs through your torso in the front, then to the legs and then back up through the spine or back. It makes a figure-eight shape. In this pattern, as your energy expands, you become part of the universe.

You do this as an individual. That is what the great Taoist masters did. It is done inside your own being and then it expands. The goal is easy to attain if you educate your spirit and soul. If you are able to do this, it will help keep you healthy. The more chi you have, the more chi you can produce. It is that simple. You need to train your mind so you can keep the chi ball alive and going. You must focus on your own personal energy and keep your mind as well as your heart paying attention to your chi. Try this with your breath. Focus on your breathing and then hold your breath. With focus you will be able to maintain more oxygen. Remember that breathing entails exhalation of carbon dioxide as well as inhaling oxygen.

Remember the various orbits. The moon is orbiting the earth, the earth is orbiting the sun, and the sun is orbiting within the galaxy (see fig. 4.7).

Also keep in mind the notable parts of the body relative to your internal orbit. Note the navel, coccyx, sacrum, lumbar, spine, and inter-

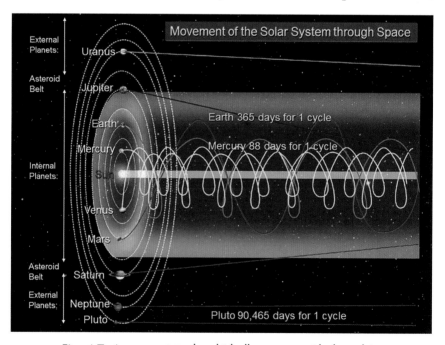

Fig. 4.7. As you rotate the chi ball, connect with the orbits
of the moon, earth, sun, and solar system.

nal chi ball orbiting with your body. Your head is moving, as are your eyes. See your Hua Hin and other major points within you. At this point, light, color, and energy come to you. Feel every electron within your being affected by your environment. You are now in touch with your original operating system. Be sure to reverse the internal spinning. Also rock yourself side to side and follow this up with the Crane Neck Exercise and Turtle Neck Exercise (see fig. 4.8).

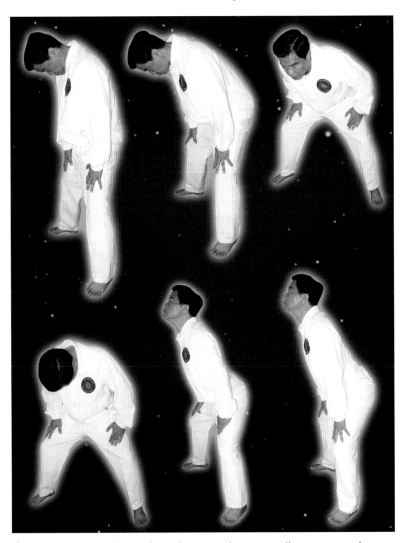

Fig. 4.8. Turtle Neck is shown in the upper illustration and Crane Neck in the lower.

Crane Neck Exercise

1. First, stretch the neck upward.
2. Next slowly bend down, essentially making a circular motion with the body while at the same time stretching outwardly. All this can be done while sitting in a chair. Keep the hands on the legs and exhale while circling the body. Make the spine soft and flexible.

 Turtle Neck Exercise

1. Put the head down with the chin on the chest, while breathing out.
2. Circle the entire body in the reverse direction as was done with the Crane Neck Exercise. The neck is tucked in tight between the shoulders. When going back up, breathe in. Lean back as the neck is pressed down.

Listen to the commands in your mind and follow them exactly. The mind, the spirit, and the heart should come together as one. Do not forget to breathe. Finally, do not forget to expand and contract as you orbit the significant parts of your body. Your awareness will increase as the planet spins around you. Once you understand the theory you can go on to practice it properly.

Connecting the Orbits

Connecting to the external orbits in the universe is as easy as taking a free ride. They are there for you and all you need to connect is the proper awareness (see figs. 4.9 and 4.10). Expand your consciousness and awaken yourself so that you are aware of the energy-creating orbits of the universe.

There are four major orbits:

1. Daily orbit
2. Monthly orbit
3. Yearly orbit
4. Largest orbit, which is the sun spinning around the galaxy

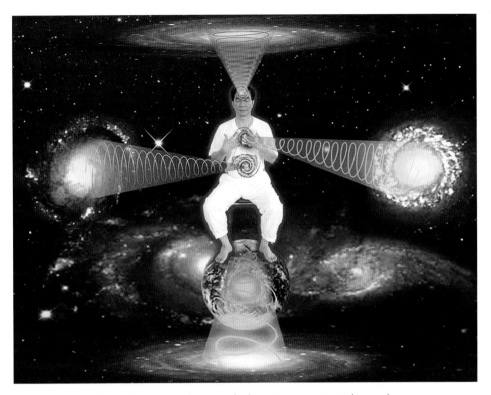

Fig. 4.9. You are born with the Microcosmic Orbit and it
connects to the orbits of the universe.

Fig. 4.10. An infinite
number of orbits
are interconnected
with your internal
Microcosmic Orbit.

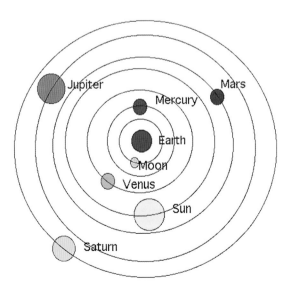

The Microcosmic Orbit will help to activate the orbiting of forces of the solar system and the universe in you by opening the flow of chi (body's life-force energy) in the energy pathways from the Hui Yin (the perineum) up the spine, through the head, and back down the front of your body. This will help to draw in more Primordial Force from the earth through the soles of the feet up to the spine and from the universe in through the crown, to combine in the lower tan tien (abdominal area), the heart, and the brain.

According to the Taoist texts, when the energy moves through the orbit we are born again. While the fetus is spinning in the mother's womb, electricity is generated. After a person is born they still have that energy. Eventually, because of imbalanced emotions or stress, it becomes depleted and blocked, making us vulnerable to sickness and disease. How quickly the energy flow can be restored depends on the individual and their understanding and training. As we know, balance is the key of the Tao. Imbalance anywhere causes serious problems or blockages.

One of the unfortunate aspects of modern life is that people do not know their own bodies. There are two things about finding balance. One is breathing. The next step is emotional balance. We all have problems of stress that affect our health and cause us to become emotionally upset. It is important that we are aware of this because accumulating more and more anger every day is very unhealthy. When we get the basics down of how to balance the body, we are healthy. Maintaining this Taoist philosophical approach prevents us from getting sick. It gives us energy. This training allows us to become wise, and through this wisdom we are able to be happy and to repair our own bodies.

This is made possible by the Microcosmic Orbit. In this meditation you let go of negative emotions into the earth energy. This will transform your negative emotions, but you have to relax and let go for it to happen. Impatience makes your heart very hot and too much heat will shake the heart, which is what a heart attack is. A tree also transforms negative energy into positive energy as it takes in carbon dioxide, our waste product, and converts it into oxygen, our food for life. Emotionally you must learn how to let go, forgive, and forget. In return you receive health, wealth, and longevity from the earth. But you need to consciously connect with the earth so it can transform your negative energy into virtuous energy.

After coming to this realization you can be more connected, more centered, and happier. Trust in and feel your Microcosmic Orbit (see fig. 4.11). Love your organs and connect them to the universal energy. Activate your Inner Smile. Your radiance and love will make the necessary connections. Feel the blessings of universal love, wisdom, and knowledge coming from the Supreme Creator or whatever Ultimate Force fits into your larger belief system. Your love is unlimited and unconditional.

Universal love starts with loving yourself and then shining the radiance to all of your internal organs. Know, feel, and love your own body. Know and experience the seasons of the year as your Microcosmic Orbit connects to the spinning of the earth by practicing these exercises daily.

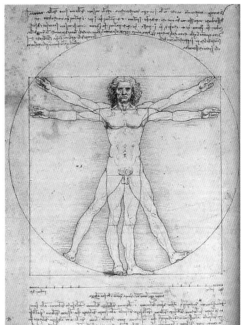

Fig. 4.11. Connect into the Universal Love (Universal Man) through your Microcosmic Orbit's natural connection to orbits of the galaxy.

Simplified Microcosmic Orbit

1. Sit with hands on knees and rock the spine. First, connect to the earth, imagining you have a long tail growing all the way down to the ground (see fig. 4.12). In the beginning you need to use mental power plus movement. The movement is essential to vibrate the coccyx. That will activate a Fire Dragon, which then spirals upward to your cranium. Feel your whole spine vibrating and feel energy come up through your spinal cord to the back of your skull.

2. Then stand up and relax the coccyx and loosen the sacrum (see fig. 4.13). Rotate the area of the sacrum in an undulating fashion. Make sure to clearly focus on this region of the body. A person that is aware enough will feel a warm sensation. Next move front to back and back to front.

3. Next sit down (see fig. 4.14). Use the index finger to touch the center of your chin and then locate the spot on top of your cranium where there was an opening at birth. With some individuals that

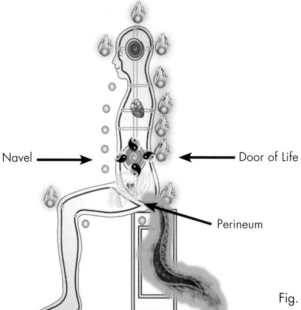

Navel

Door of Life

Perineum

Fig. 4.12. Activating the Dragon's Tail

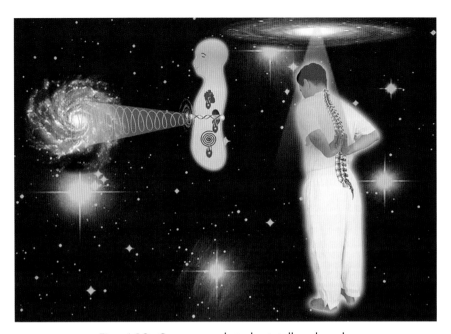

Fig. 4.13. Coccyx needs to be totally relaxed.

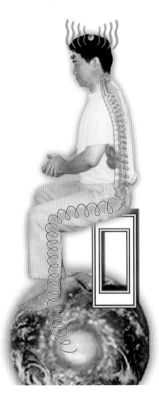

Fig. 4.14. Microcosmic Orbit
activating spine and coccyx

spot is more toward the back. Find the axis that runs from the chin to the spot on your head. That axis connects your cranium to the Big Dipper and the North Star (see fig. 4.15). Simply smile and relax upward and make the connection. Then the force can pull you upward. Relax, feeling the spine warm and relaxed.

4. Focus on the four Tai Chi balls (four directions) spinning in the lower tan tien, creating a fire chi ball.

5. Inhale with small sips (3–6 at each point) and move the fire chi ball down to Sexual Palace (located at the pubic bone), then to the Hui Yin point (perineum), and toes. Draw in gentle, cool blue earth force, then exhale.

6. Start again; inhale with small sips and move the fire chi ball into the sacrum, Door of Life (located on the spine directly opposite the navel), T11 (the eleventh thoracic vertebra, in your mid-back, opposite your solar plexus), C7 (seventh cervical vertebrae, transitioning from the thoracic region of the spine), and Jade Pillow (the back of your head between C1 and the base of the skull).

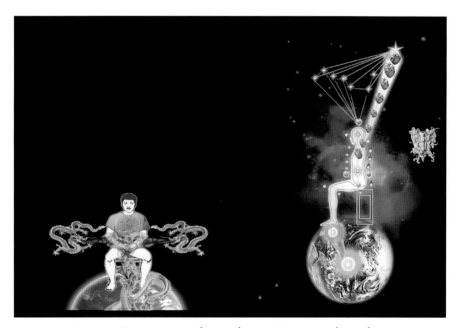

Fig. 4.15. Connecting to the earth, Big Dipper, and North Star

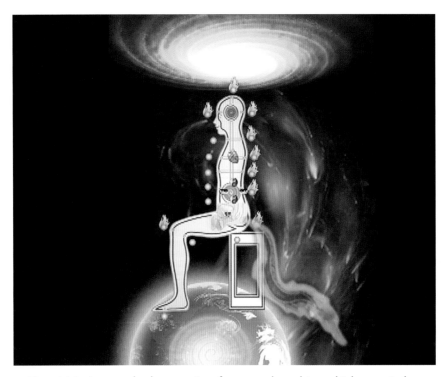

Fig. 4.16. As you do the practice, focus on the orbits, which are vital to returning to the Primordial Force.

7. Exhale then inhale (small sips) again, feeling the warm violet light of the North Star and red light of the Big Dipper directed into the crown (pineal gland).

8. Bring the spinning fire chi ball into the forehead and inhale cosmic golden light at the mid-eye.

9. With your tongue to roof of your mouth, exhale as you draw the chi down to the throat center, heart center, solar plexus, then down into the navel, breathing in and breathing out.

10. Inhale, drawing up gentle, blue earth force through the legs, perineum, spine to crown, then exhale violet red light down to mid-eye, drawing golden cosmic light down to the throat, heart, solar plexus, navel, and perineum. Do this 3 to 6 times.

11. Then collect energy at the navel and do Chi Self-Massage.

Chi Self-Massage

Simple massage techniques are used to remove blockages and to enhance the healthy distribution of chi in the body from head to toe. This is good to do after meditation and other practices where a lot of chi is activated.

The first step in this Inner Alchemy process is to feel the internal energy. The only way to understand the Tao is to feel it inside yourself. You need to feel the internal energy before you can cultivate it. That is why you should always start your daily practice with the Inner Smile. It creates the proper environment for your internal transformation. Through the Inner Smile you get in touch mentally with your five vital organs and related organs, by smiling down each line—Functional Channel (front), digestive tract (middle), and Governor Channel (back, spinal cord, and crown)—using your eyes to connect with each part of your body. By doing this on a daily basis you will start to develop a personal relationship with yourself on the physical, emotional, mental, and energetic (spiritual) levels.

By using the autonomic nervous system internally through your eyes, you generate a parasympathetic (positive) response and create a good feeling of love in your body. Your heart generates this smiling energy when you focus your eyes into your heart with positive thoughts. When you smile down your body, your body will respond with positive, loving energy. This is how we learn to generate love within ourselves instead of taking it from others; the abundance of that love within us will spread to others energetically across time and space without trying to give love to anyone.

It is like greeting someone with a handshake, hug, or smile: they will respond the same. Now, however, you do it internally to all your internal body parts, and you feel relaxed, calm, and at peace. By doing this, you create the proper internal environment to proceed with the next step in cultivating your internal energy in a systemic pattern: Chi Self-Massage.

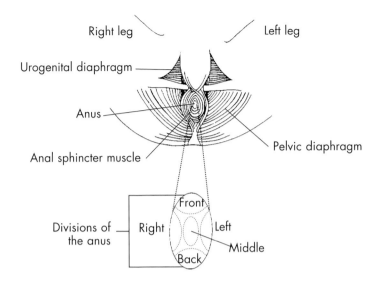

Fig. 4.17. Five regions of the anus

It is important to know the five regions of the anus, as they correspond to specific organs in the body. Contracting each specific area brings chi to its related organs (see fig. 4.17).

Simplified Chi Self-Massage

1. Rub hands and contract anus, then place palms on eyes.
2. Inhale and contract genitals, buttocks, and anus, then send energy through eyes, feet, and hands.
3. Place fingertips on eyes: rub clockwise and counterclockwise (repeat 9 times).
4. Pull out eyelids then clench fist and rub eye sockets (repeat 9 times).
5. Focus on a finger 8 inches from eyes until eyes tear.
6. Cover eyes with cupped palms and rotate them clockwise and counterclockwise (repeat 9 times).
7. Inhale and contract perineum, pull eyeballs back, exhale and release perineum (repeat 9 times).

8. Inhale and contract middle anus and middle of eyeballs; exhale and release (repeat 9 times).

9. Inhale and contract front anus and top of eyeballs; exhale and release (repeat 9 times).

10. Inhale and contract back anus and bottom of eyeballs; exhale and release (repeat 9 times).

11. Inhale and contract right anus and right of eyeballs; exhale and release (repeat 9 times).

12. Inhale and contract left anus and left of eyeballs; exhale and release (repeat 9 times).

13. Stick fingers in nostrils, then move left, right, up, and down.

14. Pinch and rub bridge of nose, then inhale and press (repeat 9 times).

15. Massage sides of nose, then rub below nose (repeat 9 times).

16. Place right fingers on Sexual Palace and left fingers on sacrum, then rotate, lift sacrum and coccyx up and down (repeat 3 times).

17. Rub front and back of ears between fingers (repeat 9 times).

18. Rub ear shells with fingers, then pull down lobes (repeat 9 times).

19. Put fingers in ears. Inhale (close anus), then exhale (repeat 9 times).

20. Pinch nostrils, then blow and swallow air, then release (repeat 3 times).

21. Cover your ears with your palms, fingers pointing toward the back of your head. In this position, flick your index fingers against your third fingers so that the index fingers drum on the lower edge (occipital bone) of the skull to vibrate and stimulate the inner ears' mechanism (repeat 9 times).

22. Open mouth and tap skin around gums with fingertips.

23. Massage gums with tongue then swallow saliva (repeat 9 times).

24. Thrust tongue out, down, and up, then curl tongue, pressing hard to palate, contracting anus and esophagus.

25. Tap teeth, then inhale and pull up anus, then swallow saliva.

26. Spread thumbs from forefingers, then wipe neck from chin down with "V" formed by thumb and forefinger, alternating hands (repeat 9 times).

27. Tap and raise shoulders up and exhale down (repeat 9 times).
28. Knuckle tap and rub scalp and temples (repeat 9 times).
29. Wipe whole face, alternating flattened fingers of each hand, first side to side, then up and down (repeat 9 times).
30. Bladder Chi Kung: sit or stand on toes, then urinate:
    a) Stop urine, then inhale and pull up on perineum, then clench teeth, pressing down on bladder.
    b) Exhale, then release urine, squeezing prostate (men) or vagina (women) (repeat 3 times).
    c) Urinate halfway, building up pressure, then release (repeat 3 times).
31. Open heart, then open eyes, then warm navel (men use right palm over navel and left palm over it; women reverse).
32. Foot massage: toe and heel stretch inward toward stomach, first right foot then left.
33. Tendon stretch: stretch fingers to toes and do bellows breathing (exhale and suck in your stomach and abdominal area until it is flat and tucked in toward your spine, then inhale until that area is inflated) (repeat 9 times), then exhale with tongue out to chin (repeat 9 times).
34. Thymus: do knuckle tapping on chest and heart, followed by light palming (9 times).
35. Lung and liver: lightly palm slap and rub (repeat 9 times).
36. Stomach, spleen, and pancreas: rub crossways (repeat 9 times).
37. Abdomen and intestines: rub in a clockwise circle (repeat 9 times).
38. Kidney backside: do fist hitting and warm palming (repeat 9 times).
39. Sacrum backside: do wrist and fist hitting on one side at a time, then both sides (repeat 9 times).
40. Knee cap: do moving massage, then behind knee slapping (repeat 9 times).
41. Foot Kidney point: spread toes, then rub soles.
42. Palm and finger: massage, activating related organs.
43. Spinal Cord Breathing: move fists in front of chest, then inhale,

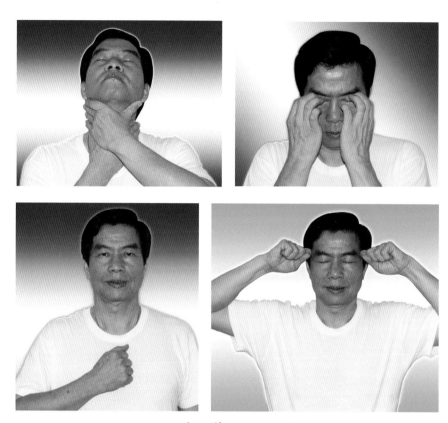

Fig. 4.18. Chi Self-Massage techniques

drawing back elbows while tilting head back with chin in; then exhale, bringing elbows, chin, and head into chest (repeat 9 times).

44. Turtle Neck: sink chin down, out, and up; then reverse and do Crane Neck (repeat 9 times).

45. Elephant swings his trunk: drop arms and inhale, swinging arms up to touch fingers at eye level, then exhale, swinging arms down, back, and forward as body rocks with feet (repeat 30 times).

Six Healing Sounds

The Universal Healing Tao system is a safe, practical way to work with your internal energy. When you work with internal energy you create

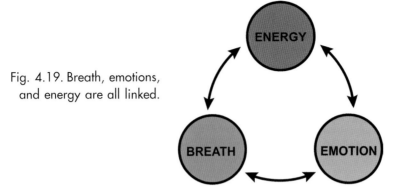

Fig. 4.19. Breath, emotions, and energy are all linked.

heat. Six Healing Sounds is the last formula you do in your daily practice because this Inner Alchemy practice cools the energy down. Once you learn the Inner Smile and the Six Healing Sounds you can safely add any or all of the 240 plus formulas of the Universal Healing Tao system. You start with the Inner Smile and end your daily practice with the Six Healing Sounds. They are also great at bedtime.

The lungs' sound is the first. Each sound is done following the same pattern: you inhale and look into the organ and locate any negative emotions residing there (for the lungs, the negative emotions are sadness and grief). As you exhale, you look right and left, which deletes the negative emotions from your lungs and any links to them in the brain; the negative emotions are composted and recycled in the earth (see fig. 4.19). You relax and let go. Then you do the sound again and breathe in the positive emotions of that organ and the light connected with them (for the lungs it is white light and courage, righteousness, and justice).

The Healing Sounds help you to let go of pain and suffering. You can release everything, because the earth is capable of taking on our negativity and pain. If we have difficulty understanding this, we need only to think of composting. When we compost leftover food or even the excrement of living creatures, Mother Earth turns that into something positive. And, in fact, without such recycling, she would begin to lose her energy.

Simplified Six Healing Sounds

1. Breathe in slowly and deeply, being aware of lungs. Raise arms up to eye level, rotate palms down, and raise them above head. Very slowly blow out dark murky color, excess heat, sick energy of sadness and depression, while making the lungs' sound: sss-s-s-s-s-s.

   Breathe in pure white light and transform it to courage. Float palms down to lungs, then to lap (palms up); close eyes, smiling to lungs; experience the feelings of courage and justice grow within you. Repeat 3–6 times.

2. Breathe in slowly and deeply, being aware of kidneys, then bend forward, clasp hands, close legs, and hook hands around knees. Then pull back to kidneys and look up. Breathe out very dark murky color, wet sick energy of fear, while making the kidneys' sound: choo-oo-oo-oo.

   Breathe in bright blue energy and transform it to gentleness. sitting up with open legs and palms to kidneys. Close eyes, smiling to kidneys, with palms to lap, experiencing gentleness and stillness. Repeat 3–6 times.

3. Breathe in slowly and deeply, being aware of the liver. Swing arms out overhead, clasping hands, then push palm heels right while bending slightly left. Look up. Very slowly breathe out dark murky color, excess heat, anger, aggression, while making the liver's sound: sh-h-h-h-h-h.

   Breathe in bright green energy and transform it to kindness. Unclasp hands and palms, cover liver, then move your hands to lap with palms up; close eyes, smiling down to liver. Experience kindness within you. Repeat 3–6 times.

4. Breathe in slowly and deeply, being aware of the heart. Swing arms out overhead, clasping hands, then push palm heels left while bending slightly right. Look up. Very slowly breathe out dark murky color, excess heat, cruelty, and hatred, while making the heart's sound: haw-w-w-w-w-w.

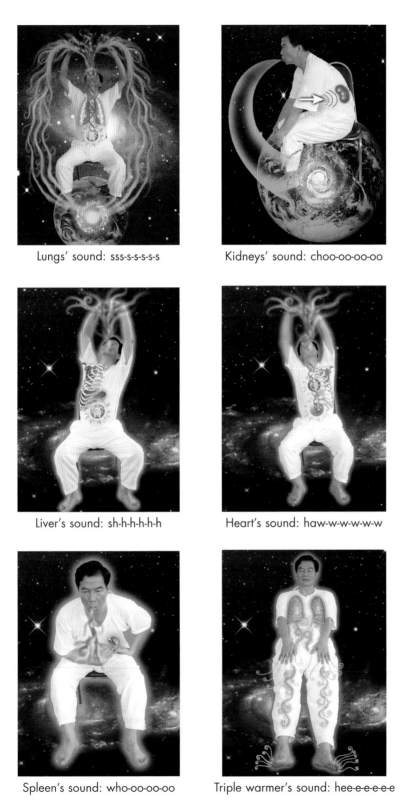

Lungs' sound: sss-s-s-s-s-s

Kidneys' sound: choo-oo-oo-oo

Liver's sound: sh-h-h-h-h

Heart's sound: haw-w-w-w-w-w

Spleen's sound: who-oo-oo-oo

Triple warmer's sound: hee-e-e-e-e

Fig. 4.20. Six Healing Sounds

Breathe in bright red energy and transform it to joy, love, and respect. Unlock hands, cover heart with palms, then move your hands to lap, with palms up; close eyes, smiling to heart and feeling the joy, love, happiness, patience, and respect growing within you. Repeat 3–6 times.

5. Breathe in slowly and deeply, being aware of the spleen. Swing arms around, placing fingers below left of sternum; press in, pushing out middle back. Very slowly breathe out a dark murky color, excess heat, dampness, worry, anxiety, while making the spleen's sound: who-oo-oo-oo.

Breathe in bright yellow light and transform it to fairness, balance, and openness. Sit up with palms over spleen then move hands to lap. Close eyes, smiling down to spleen, and experience fairness, openness, and centering growing within your body. Repeat 3–6 times.

6. Lie on your back, then close eyes and move hands down your sides. Breathe in and feel the expansion of the upper (brain, heart, lungs), middle (liver, kidneys, stomach, pancreas, and spleen), and lower (large and small intestines, bladder, and sexual organs) energy centers, and hold.

Then breathe out from upper, middle, and lower, while making triple warmer's sound: hee-e-e-e-e. Empty and hold, then breathe normally. Smile. Rest and feel light and empty. Repeat 3–6 times.

Simplified Simple Chi Kung

1. Knock on the Door of Life area with your fists from rib cage down to sacrum, breathing deeply into lower back (9 times).
2. Legs and Hips: Shift weight from foot to foot and drop your body lower and lower with feet flat and waist straight (9 times).
3. Knees: Feet together and rotate knees with hands (counterclockwise 9 times).
4. Shoulders: Stretch from fingertips extending arms (3 times).
   a) Arms Down: Shoulders to ears. Hold, back, and drop.

b) Arms Forward: Shoulders to ears. Hold, back, and drop.

c) Arms Up: Shoulders to ears. Hold, back, and drop.

d) Arms to Sides: Shoulders to ears. Hold, back, and drop.

5. Neck: Rotate head with eyes to sides, up and down.

6. Tai Chi Chi Kung Warm Ups:

  a) Standing Posture, arms at sides and turn hips side to side. Relax spine and let arms swing naturally (9 times) (see fig. 4.21 on page 168).

  b) Opening Door of Life: Draw right arm up to eyes across torso to left with palm facing away while left arm swings over Door of Life (opposite navel) reaching fully. Relax and extend lower back, stretching each time, then reverse to right and repeat steps (9 times on each side).

  c) Bouncing: Open joints and bounce body up and down gently, vibrating hanging arms but feet do not leave ground (30 times).

  d) Leg Kicking: Center sacrum over right heel and raise left leg and right arm and gently kick out, then reverse (30 times).

  e) Rotate ankle, knee, and hips each time the same way (3 times).

7. Windmill:

  a) Outer Front Extension: Widen stance and hook thumbs and hands close to torso. Inhale, raising arms over head, extending spine backward. Exhale slowly, bending forward, stretching down lumbar, thoracic, and cervical vertebrae, and slowly move palms up body front (3 times).

  b) Inner Front Extension: Reverse, pointing fingertips down to torso, activating vertebrae with arms out and up (3 times).

  c) Left Outer Extension: Arms over head, turn shoulders left, then lean back to right and move down left side across lower front to right side and up. Lean back to left, turning shoulders to right, and lean back to right (3 times).

  d) Right Outer Extension: Reverse, turning shoulders to right, leaning back to left, then down right across front left and up, then back to right, turning shoulders left and down (3 times).

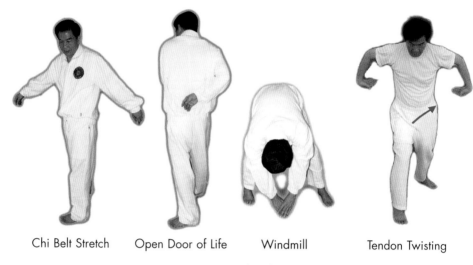

Chi Belt Stretch   Open Door of Life   Windmill   Tendon Twisting

Fig. 4.21. Simple Chi Kung

8. Tendon Twisting: Reach forward, twisting arms out in circles and return (3 times), then reverse (3 times). Do sides, top, and bottom then do a larger circle series (3 times each).

9. Lower Back Stretches (lie on stomach):
   a) Hands under shoulders and push shoulders up (20 times).
   b) Tighten back, head up, hands on buttocks, and squeeze each buttock 6 times. Do 10 sets.
   c) Tighten back, head up, and grab wrists over back, then squeeze, tightening lower back (20 times).
   d) Tighten back, head up, connecting fingers on back of head, and turn to right and left (10 times).
   e) Tighten back, head up, connecting fingers on back of head, and lift elbows up right then left (10 times).
   f) Tighten back, head up, drawing hands overhead, then down to buttocks, swinging from side to side (10 times).
   g) Turn over on back, head down, and shake arms and legs in air, detoxifying organs, to 60 counts.
   h) Draw heels to buttocks and draw knees together, moving them up and down (60 times).

Cosmic Nutrition

To improve our health, we need to start listening to our bodies, seeing where the imbalances lie and finding the ways to restore balance to them. Rather than just applying the same dietary therapy to all people, Cosmic Nutrition offers ways of observing and measuring yin and yang imbalances and then using five-element therapy to restore health.

LIVING TAO (EMOTIONAL BODY): INTERMEDIATE PRACTICES

Laughing Chi Kung

One of the first things we must learn is that we are responsible for our emotions, our psychological state, and everything about us. This includes our body and our health. We can hire lawyers, doctors, accountants, and psychologists, but that never changes who we are. That is what the Tao teaches us. We know our own bodies because we are the only ones who can feel what is inside us. And we actually know how to fix ourselves. We know our life and the people in it.

Metaphorically, we know our internal army, an enormous army of white blood cells that protects us from disease. The soldiers in our body need training and maintenance just like any army does. We cannot expect untrained soldiers to fight a war. We must remember to train the soldiers every day through our Taoist practices. One way to train our soldiers is to laugh. Among the numerous things that this accomplishes is activating the thymus. Our thymus, or little heart, is right in the middle of the chest.

If we look inward, we can see the white blood cells marching to the thymus when we laugh. There they become the soldiers that heal and protect us. They fight for us against viruses and cancer. Ordinary cells will not kill handicapped cells because, metaphorically speaking, they are brothers and sisters. Only special killer cells will do the job. We can think of the abdomen and the small intestine as a big training camp where antibodies are trained to go to war against disease and imbalance. The liver and the spleen enter to help with the training, but the abdomen is the biggest training camp. As the blood flows naturally through the abdomen, a program is injected and antibodies are created. This program allows the antibodies to recognize all the different types of bacteria.

You can train these cells with a deep and long-lasting belly laugh. Emphasize the abdomen. Then rub the navel and abdominal wall. Visualize small soldiers marching into the intestinal tissues. You will feel warmth developing. Laughing is a kind of organ self massage (see fig. 4.22). Each day with this practice, you accumulate more and more happiness.

We have talked about the war within the body, but at the same time love is happening in the body. There is what can be thought of as cellular love, and that is the process that creates new cells in our body. Love

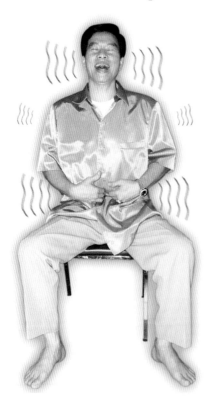

Fig. 4.22. The power of laughter

makes us happy. We can build up our level of happiness little by little and one day at a time. While it is true that stress is a serious problem, particularly in the modern world, we have the natural equipment to solve problems: specifically, our minds and our bodies. The more problems we have, the more experience we gain, and ultimately this means that we will have fewer problems. The end result of this is the acquisition of wisdom.

Elixir Chi Kung

Saliva is known as the elixir of life because of the alchemical power contained in water. This practice activates the saliva and charges it with oxygen and the chi of nature, earth, and the cosmos. With the Elixir Swallow technique, the charged saliva is turned into instant chi (life force)—the most powerful healing power. The procedure for Elixir Chi Kung is to first swish your saliva around in your mouth from left to right and up and down. Do this thoroughly and completely. This allows oxygenation of the substance as you blend it with all the hormones and various essences found in the mouth to make the special nectar. You go on to consciously massage your gums with your tongue. This strengthens them because of the power of the elixir.

Without swallowing, you then visualize a scene in nature that inspires you, such as a mountain stream, a beautiful beach with crystal clear water, or a riverside view of a pristine landscape, while you spread your arms as if embracing nature itself. When you breathe and contract your anus, the suction in your abdomen will draw up the energy of Mother Earth and activate your third eye and crown. You can then begin to experience transcendence as your awareness expands outward to embrace the cosmos. Still without swallowing, you take in the chi as you chew your saliva. After pressing on your palate with your tongue, you finally swallow the chi-enhanced saliva and concentrate on your tan tien and the area around your navel at the same time. You will feel the power in your body as you believe and experience the essence of the universal force.

Activate Three Tan Tiens

 ## Simplified Opening Three Fires and Three Tan Tiens

1. Smile down your shoulders and palms into ground, lifting index fingers up and drawing up earth energy.
2. Move palms in front of lower tan tien, opening tan tien fire. Feel fire burning and the warmth spreading throughout body.
3. Move palms to Ming Men, opening kidney fire. Feel fire burning and the warmth spreading up to and filling the brain.
4. Move palms to sternum, opening heart fire. Feel fire burning and the warmth spreading up into brain.

Connect with the Six Directions

This powerful energetic technique teaches you how to expand your mind and chi, to touch the force in the cosmos, and to draw that energy back into the body. By practicing the Six Directions daily you will increase your healing and cosmic power. It begins with the Three Minds into One practice.

 ## Three Minds into One

1. Relax the body by smiling down.
2. Empty the mind down: turn the upper mind into an observing mind, and observe inwardly; fuse three minds into one mind at the lower tan tien and keep it spiraling.
3. Expand the spiraling chi to the mid-eyebrow, crown, and forehead, and thence into the universe.

You then expand into the six directions, below, above, front, back, left, and right, and feel yourself being charged by the universe from all

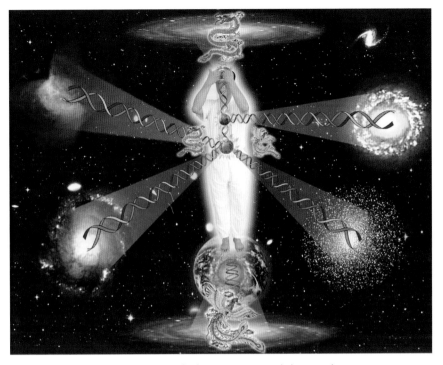

Fig. 4.23. Connect with the universe and the six directions.

six directions (see fig. 4.23). The ancient Taoists associated directions with different animals. The white tiger is to the right or the west. The green dragon is to the left or the east. The red pheasant is to the south, in front of you, or on the top. The turtle or black warrior is in the north or at your back or on the feet. Finally, in the center or on the top is the phoenix. These animals are our protectors and are intelligent entities. They protect us from evil (negative energy) and guide us safely.

Tao Yin

Tao Yin is a Taoist yoga that stimulates chi flow in particular meridians (chi pathways delineated in the acupuncture maps of the energy body in traditional Chinese medicine). Tao Yin coordinates deep breathing, chi, mind, and body for deep sensing, helping you to be more relaxed and refreshed. It induces elasticity of tendons, ligaments, and associated muscles, and conditions the spine, psoas muscles, and patterns of movement for health and inner development.

Simplified Tao Yin Practices

Lying on your back, place palms on the following areas and breathe into palms (6 times each):

1. Abdomen (navel area)
2. Upper abdomen (stomach area)
3. Lower abdomen (tan tien—bladder area)
4. Groin (both sides)
5. Right palm on sacrum, turn head right and left on Jade Pillow
6. Sides of chi belt (sides above hips)
7. Kidneys (lower back)
8. Diaphragm (liver and spleen)
9. Lower lungs (lower rib cage)
10. Upper lungs (upper rib cage)
11. Scapulae (cross arms and palms on upper back)
12. Neck (cross hands and palms on sides of neck)
13. Temple (sides of head)
14. Crown (both palms on top of head)
15. Whole body (palms down at sides)

Now do the Fanning technique with the haw-w-w-w-w-w sound to clear the Heart meridian. Put feet to buttocks and raise sacrum (palms at sides). With your legs straight, turn feet in and tighten body, then release.

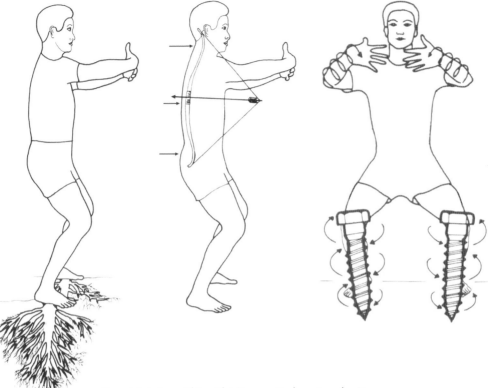

Fig. 4.24. Iron Shirt Chi Kung—Embracing the Tree

Iron Shirt Chi Kung

Iron Shirt Chi Kung enables you to build an Iron Shirt body by using the Iron Shirt packing technique while in six specific postures. In this practice Packing Process Breathing is combined with rooting to the ground, which helps to unify and strengthen bone structure alignment. It is a way of circulating the forces of the earth and the universe.

Iron Shirt Chi Kung includes the following exercises: Embracing the Tree (see fig. 4.24), Holding the Golden Urn, Turtle, Water Buffalo, and Golden Phoenix.

Simplified Iron Shirt Chi Kung Practices

1. Do lower abdominal breathing softly and slowly (9–18 times).

2. Exhale, flattening stomach and lower diaphragm. Inhale. Tighten perineum and anus, pulling up with small sips front, middle, back, left, and right anus, then genitals, then pack right and left kidneys, spiraling into navel (9 times in, 9 times out). Inhale into upper, middle, and lower abdomen, then perineum, expanding and forming chi ball and hold. Exhale through legs and feet (6 inches) into earth.

3. Inhale. Tighten perineum, press into ground and claw toes, then spiral soles (9 times in, 9 times out). Inhale to knees (lock knees) and perineum (9 times). Exhale into ground. Do sole, palm, and Bone Breathing.

4. Inhale (small sips) to tilted sacrum. Spiral (9 times in, 9 times out) and pack. Inhale pressing out T11 inflating kidneys forming chi belt then spiral (9 times in, 9 times out). Inhale into C7 (neck), Jade Pillow, clench teeth and squeeze skull bones and left and right brains and spiral (9 times in, 9 times out).

5. Inhale to crown (Crystal Room), becoming aware of violet red light from above, spiral (9 times in, 9 times out). Exhale (tongue up to palate) drawing down through mid-eye to solar plexus and spiral (9 times in, 9 times out), then do Microcosmic Orbit.

6. Do Bone Breathing: Absorb golden cosmic energy (5–10 minutes). Feel like a feather letting chi flow, rocking spine slightly.

7. Palms above head and gather energy, then draw down palms to navel and feet together. Collect energy at navel. Shake out.

Here is how to understand the effects of the Iron Shirt Chi Kung practice: if you take an egg and put it into an air-filled balloon and place that inside another air-filled balloon, then place it into a third air-filled balloon, then throw it against a wall, the egg will not break. The air-filled balloons are buffers for the egg. The egg is our vital organs, the air is the chi pressure enhanced by small inhalations, and the balloons are the connective issue (fascia) around the vital organs.

Tan Tien Chi Kung

Tan Tien Chi Kung cultivates and condenses chi power in all nine areas of the tan tien and the associated organs, kuas (area formed by the sacrum, groin area, hip joints, and hip flexors), tendons, and ligaments using the Dragon and Tiger Breath, and eleven animal exercise postures. By activating the Empty Force and Perineum Power with the Dragon and Tiger Breaths you create chi pressure in the body. When we get older we lose air pressure and we slowly deflate, just as a car tire loses air. Very old people look like a deflated balloon, with no bounce or buoyancy. The years of wear and tear and gravity on the body cause leakages in the body. Tan Tien Chi Kung helps to restore our air pressure, which gives our bodies form, structure, and the constitution that we need for the vitality to live our lives with zest and joy.

Tai Chi Chi Kung

These practices develop the inner structure and chi flow; they are meditation in movement, movement in meditation. Once you learn the form, which is the ten-thousand-practice rule (you do it 10,000 times), you know it completely, having activated your molecular memory. Then you do not know if you did it or if you did not do it, because it has become a meditation and has become a part of you. At that point you will have built up a complete defense system energetically through the practice with its postures and strikes (Ward Off, Rollback, Press, Push, Single Whip, and Single-Hand Push) with your muscle memory.

Stem Cell Chi Kung

With the use of a bamboo hitter and a wire hitter, parts of the body are vibrated, sending a message to the stem cells about where to go for healing and regeneration.

LIVING TAO (EMOTIONAL BODY): ADVANCED PRACTICES

Tendon Nei Kung

This is a set of eight postures to activate and grow the tendons. In them, you exhale your breath into your tan tien, close your genitals, pinch your elbows, and contract your heart (like a clenching fist) and, at the same time, torque your toes, heels, ankles, legs, hips, vertebrae, Jade Pillow, arms, and fingers with the rhythm of the earth and your heartbeat. Then you release the air pressure. As you inhale, your heart expands and your tendons release your whole body, while it effortlessly moves back to its original position by itself.

Bone Marrow Nei Kung

The Bone Marrow Nei Kung practices generate the bone marrow and activate the stem cells for regeneration and healing. The bone marrow is stimulated by hitting your bones (Wire and Rattan Hitting techniques), breathing into your bones (Bone Breathing and Compression techniques) (see fig. 4.25), and expanding, strengthening, and growing your bone marrow through genital massage and lifting (Sexual Chi Massage and Chi Weight Lifting techniques). In addition to regrowing bone marrow and strengthening the bones, these ancient mental and physical Taoist techniques are used to rejuvenate the organs and glands.

 ## Simplified Bone Marrow Nei Kung—Bone Breathing and Compression

Press fingertips and toe tips with fingernail.

1. Raise hands. Lightly pull up genitals and anus, sinking elbows. Palms down and inhale into index finger, then all fingers individu-

ally, then entire hand, feeling warm energy pass through fingertips and knuckles. Hold. Exhale. Rest hand.

2. Inhale through wrist, forearm, ulna, and radius bones. Hold each section, feeling bones expand. Exhale.

3. Inhale expanding into scapulae and C7 (neck point and head). Hold base of skull, tongue to palate, then exhale, drawing energy down to navel. Rest and absorb the chi.

4. Follow same procedure inhaling into bones of toes, feet, lower leg (tibia and fibula), thigh, and sacrum. Exhale.

5. Inhale into both hands and feet simultaneously up to shoulders and

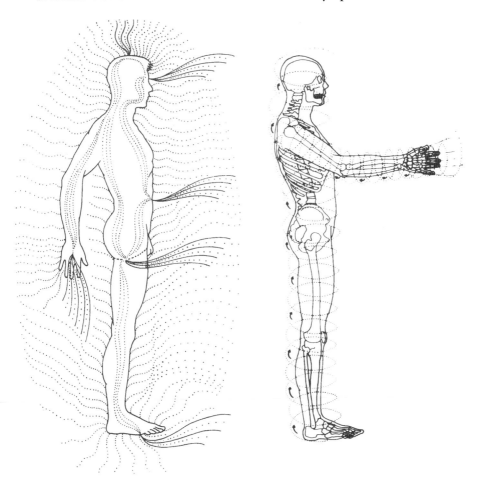

Fig. 4.25. Bone Marrow Nei Kung—Bone Breathing and Compression

scapulae through arms, then up to thigh and hip bones through legs. Hold. Exhale. Relax.

6. Inhale in sacrum through spine to T11 simultaneously with shoulders to C7 into cranial bones, down facial and collarbones, spreading through ribs to sternum. Hold, then exhale.

7. Inhale, spiral, pack, and squeeze into hands, arms, shoulders, scapulae, and collarbones through spine and T11. Hold and exhale.

8. Follow same procedure into feet, legs, hip, sacrum, and T11.

9. Inhale, spiral, pack, and squeeze into T11, spine, neck, and cranium with tongue to palate, clenching teeth. Hold and exhale.

10. Inhale, spiral, pack, and squeeze each of ribs, compressing them into sternum. Sink chest squeezing muscles. Exhale.

11. After each inhalation and exhalation, pause for 5 to 10 minutes and feel bones expand and contract with each breath.

12. Advanced: Do whole procedure, combining lower and upper together in one breath, growing the bones and bone marrow.

Tai Chi Fa Jin

This higher level of moving meditation uses the discharge technique to absorb and transmit the universal and earth forces. Through the Tai Chi Fa Jin form you learn how the discharge power is revealed through the practice of the Discharge Form and technical exercises.

Tai Chi Wu Style

Unlike the Yang form, the Wu style of eight directions is characteristically performed in a small frame in a high stance. Your daily practice of the Tai Chi forms enforces their movements in your energy body, the body that you travel with to the next realm. It teaches anatomical and geographical placement of the body, chi movements that open up your tendons and expand your body strength with the spirit aspects of the form.

CHI NEI TSANG (PHYSICAL BODY): BASIC PRACTICES

Basic Chi Nei Tsang

Chi Nei Tsang is the most powerful massage therapy for deep organ detoxification. It removes physical and emotional blockages to return body systems to healthy functioning. Each organ contains part of the Primordial Force. When an organ's accumulated negative emotions and toxins are released, the organ can more effectively draw in the Primordial Force and regenerate itself.

Cosmic Detox

The seemingly healthy person must first pass through a condition of cleansing or sickness, so to speak, or at least an intermediary stage of sickness, before attaining the higher level of health. Cosmic Detox is the regulation of human health through our diet, and most importantly, through limiting it, and through regular cleansing of the body's nine openings.

CHI NEI TSANG (PHYSICAL BODY): ADVANCED PRACTICES

Advanced Chi Nei Tsang

More techniques are taught and powerful applications are applied to release deep tension in blocked tissues. The magic of the elbow is learned to aid healing. The emotions and winds accumulate in the abdominal and navel area of the body and Advanced Chi Nei Tsang teaches you how to release the bad winds and sweep them out to reestablish a healthy flow (good winds) of vital energy. This gives you a new approach to healing by understanding the origin of the winds and the problems they create in the body, and then health can be restored.

Chi Nei Ching

Good health depends on the free flow of life-force energy, chi, throughout the entire body. The accumulation of tensions in the muscles and tendons, as well as the stagnation of negative energy, can lead to blockages in the body's energy channels, resulting in pain, low energy, or illness. Chi Nei Ching includes detailed massage techniques for unblocking chi, releasing tight tendons and muscles, and alleviating back and joint pain.

Karsai Nei Tsang

This genital health therapeutic cleansing massage specifically improves the health of the genitals and the genital area. The massage movements break up and dissolve sedimentation in the circulatory system, release toxicity, and remove physical and emotional blockages in the pelvic

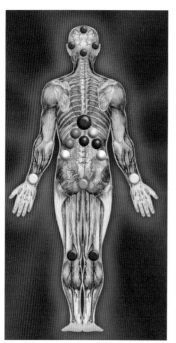 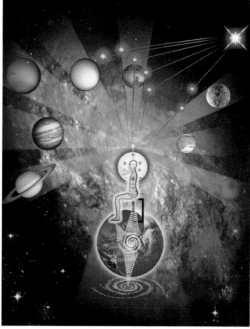

Fig. 4.26. Chi Nei Tsang (physical body) and
Cosmic Healing (energy body)

area. Most recipients experience a strong sensation of opening of the energy channels from the sexual area to the kidneys, abdomen, legs, the brain, and other parts of the body. This enables the Primordial Force and the stem cells to refresh, heal, and regenerate more effectively in these areas as well as in the local sexual area.

Life Pulse Massage

Blood and chi often flow side by side throughout the body, the blood acting as the vehicle for our vital energy. Areas of slow or congested circulation lead to blockages in the flow of vital energy and toxin accumulation in the body. The practice of Life Pulse Massage allows these blockages to be cleared, revitalizing cardiovascular function, detoxifying the organs, and restoring the flow of blood and chi throughout the body.

COSMIC HEALING (ENERGY BODY): BASIC PRACTICES

The basic practices of Cosmic Healing enhance your connection to the cosmos. Taoist Cosmic Chi Kung introduces basic practices for general healing sessions with specific light energies of the Primordial Force. The procedure for creating healing "chi" water by changing the water's structure with one's mind-eye-heart power and Primordial Force is also taught.

COSMIC HEALING (ENERGY BODY): INTERMEDIATE PRACTICES

Taoist Astral Healing

More advanced methods are learned, and specific healing applications are taught for specific ailments in specific areas of the body. The practitioner learns meditations focused on connecting parts of the body to the structure of the universe in the process of spiritualization and opening to more powerful healing experiences with the Primordial Force.

Wisdom Chi Kung

 ## Simplified Wisdom Chi Kung

In Wisdom Chi Kung you feed your brain with the cosmos (see fig. 4.27).

1. Smile down and empty mind, filling abdomen brain with chi.

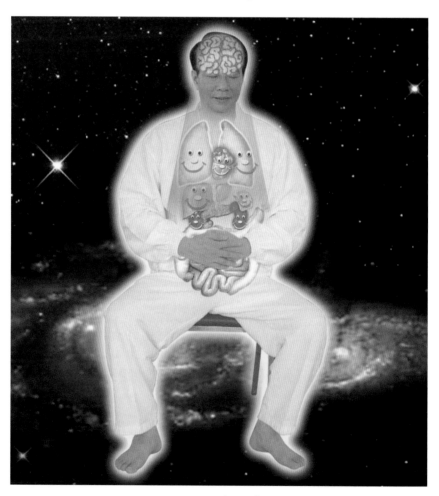

Fig. 4.27. Wisdom Chi Kung

2. Activate tan tien fire and kidney fires, retaining 95 percent aware-ness at tan tien, drawing in cosmic energy.

3. Activate heart fire (imperial fire), creating softness and joy.

4. Smile down to kidneys and feel blue chi rise, filling back of brain, left and right, then sexual organs (center of brain).

5. Smile down, filling right brain with green liver energy, front center brain with red heart energy, left brain with yellow spleen energy, and right and left front brain with white lung energy, growing brain with vital organ rainbow colors.

6. With brain filled with rainbow chi, connect with star above.

7. Smile and completely empty brain to stars and galaxies.

8. Expand good intentions to universal energies and the energy will return multiplied to fill the brain with wisdom.

9. Empty brain again to universe, filling the brain again with universal life force, wisdom, knowledge, and understanding.

Sun, Moon, Tree, Star Chi Kung

 ## Simplified Sun, Moon, Tree, Star Practices

1. Look, blinking, at sun, then close eyes and breathe in violet, red, and yellow colors at mid-eye, into your senses and cells (6 times).

2. Feel the sun's colored rays move down body into your bones with a cosmic baptism, as organ colors start to glow with sun.

3. Smile at moon, opening mouth, and draw in moon silver essence, mixing with your saliva (sticky honey taste), and swallow down to navel (6 times), feeling silver light absorb into body. Do orbits.

4. Extend palms, facing tree, focusing at nose tip, using eyes to guide tree energy inside your left arm to crown and back through right palm into tree, letting tree flow come back (18 times).

5. Move tree energy inside arms to crown and down Functional Channel to feet (10 feet) into ground, then up into tree trunk and up to tree top, then down your body and reverse (36 times).

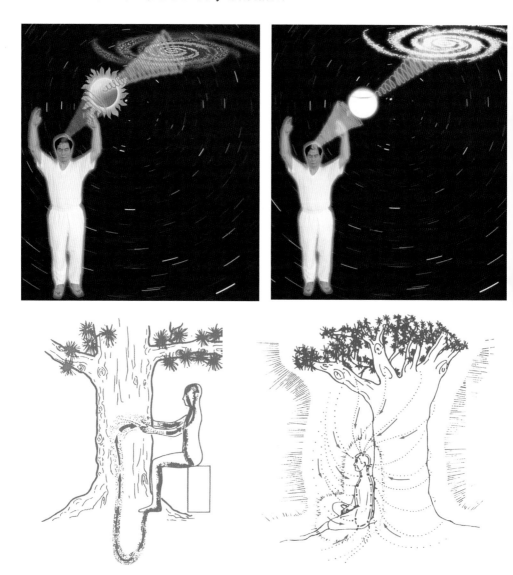

Fig. 4.28. Sun, Moon, and Tree Chi Kung

6. Connect skull points with Big Dipper and North Star to Dubhe (purple and cerebellum), Merak (dark blue and memory), Phecda (light blue and pineal), Megrez (green and thalamus), Alioth (yellow and pituitary), Mizar (orange and olfactory), and Alcor (red and third eye).

Sexual Alchemy

The Taoist system of transforming sexual energy is very practical and flexible. It does not require gurus or priests; it just requires you, and a trust in the Tao and its concept and theory, along with the practices in the Universal Healing Tao. It is good to know and study other religions and to have a grasp of their systems. One thing you should always watch for is whether or not they have a formula or steps that can be done by anyone. The Tao teaches that every person has a channel to God, Heaven, the Original Force, and the cosmos. The Taoist practices of Sexual Alchemy presented here are ancient and have helped many on their journey, not just to happiness but to the sublime oneness of the universe. Enlightenment or self-realization is up to you and you alone.

A key of the Universal Healing Tao practice has to do with understanding sexual energetic practices. One point to realize is that for a man too much sex in the form of ejaculations begins to drain the energy in the kidneys. If this happens, the body begins to draw the energy from the brain. There is almost a chain reaction, because the next thing that is drawn upon is the heart or perhaps the lungs. Comprehending this is the start to having the wisdom of the ancient Taoist masters. Every day cells break down and you need fresh cells to replace them. This means DNA renewal. The exercises and concepts

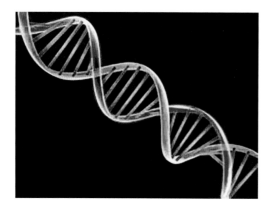

Fig. 5.1. DNA has the ability to split, make love, and create another cell.

in this book are designed to initiate you into the circle of wisdom of the ancient Taoist masters.

When you feel sexual arousal or want to make love, this is mirrored in your DNA. The DNA itself also feels arousal and goes on to make love as well. When your DNA makes love it creates another cell replete with Original Force just as your body itself has this quality. When your parents made love they passed this on to you. Thus the entire cycle of the creation of life and energy is involved in this theory. Your parents experienced love, joy, and happiness and made love. By doing this they passed on the love, joy, and happiness within them directly to their child. Studies have shown that during sexual arousal the sperm itself vibrates and the hair on the woman's egg vibrates as well. This creates a lot of chi. Love, arousal, and orgasm are the basic energies of your cells. Every cell needs these qualities.

Orgasm takes place in a short amount of time and consequently people want more. Each time that a man ejaculates, his sexual energy is diminished, but there is a way to multiply orgasms so you will not use up your sexual energy. For both men and women, the solution is to have orgasms but to use them to accomplish a state of bliss. There are many people claiming to be able to help others reach a state of bliss, but the secret is within. This is also the healing power of the ancient sages and entails causing the DNA to split in a healthy manner.

The place to start is with collecting the energy. This is similar to the fundamental principle of economics, which states that in order to make money you must first save money. Money is of no use to the body, but energy is. Storing energy is a sign of great wisdom. If you do not store the energy correctly, too much energy remains in the head or the heart. The heart is pulsing continuously, creating heat. Science tells us that everything that moves generates heat and has the potential to become extremely hot. There is a great deal of heat in the brain as well. Years ago, in the early stages of the computer age, scientists said that in order to replicate the functions of the human brain a computer would have to be enormous; bigger than the Empire State Building. However, even if such a computer could be built, there would be a problem cooling it. They surmised that in order to cool it, a second structure the same size would be required.

Your brain cannot store energy and neither can your heart. The brain can send energy and receive energy. That is the function of your brain as well as your heart. In addition, your heart has a specialized function; namely, it can multiply energy. The tan tien can store a vast amount of energy that comes in through the head and the heart. True happiness must not be something so hot that you burn up. Wisdom is required to have actual and meaningful happiness because it has its own cooling system. Wisdom comes slowly so you do not set yourself on fire and destroy yourself.

The training of the Universal Healing Tao system prevents overheating. Your energy can be transformed into chi based on the principle of $E = mc^2$. The principle is this simple: have trust and then utilize the natural energy of your body to create chi. Then communicate with the Original Force. Trust means you have the ability to use the heart energy and the chi within you for transformation. This requires time and patience. Discipline is necessary to acquire good chi. This chi changes and transforms, allowing great energy to flow when you massage your breasts and genitals and transmit the healing power within you. Your body has continuous combustion and this affects the chi in your body.

Chi moves everything and is like electricity. You can think of it as a battery that you need to keep charged. All of your energy can be guided into your organs to revitalize them.

You can recognize and activate the inner connections of your body by doing important practices such as breastfeeding, laughing, and utilizing the Inner Smile. With the interconnection of internal organs, breastfeeding activates the thymus and the spleen. This helps prevent damage to the cells of your body that have the potential of becoming cancerous (see fig. 5.2).

A woman's breasts swell each month before menstruation; they are preparing nutrition to make milk because the ovaries are ready to produce a baby. When nothing happens, everything is cleaned out with the blood. However, instead of being discarded, this vital energy can actually be used to create extra energy. If you are a woman you need to know that it is important to keep the breasts young and supple or the milk will go bad, get stuck, and eventually cause a tumor.

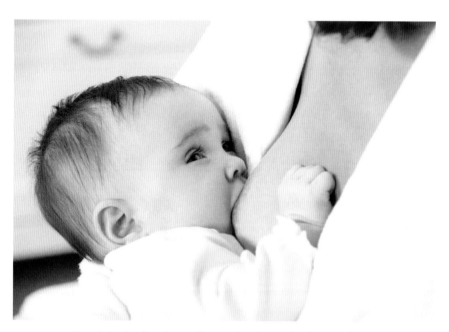

Fig. 5.2. Studies have shown that breastfeeding reduces
the chance of getting breast cancer.

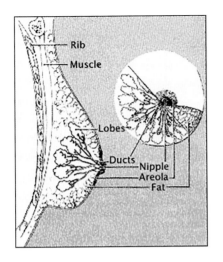

Fig. 5.3. The breasts and uterus are important in creating cancer-fighting cells in a woman's body.

Consequently, breast massage is of great importance to health. More and more medical professionals encourage massage of the breasts. The nipple should be pinched so that there is a connection to the uterus. These two things are also closely connected to sexual activity. This means that your uterus and ovaries are the first connection if you are a woman (see fig. 5.3).

Men also have this ability, but not to the degree that women do. With men the breasts are connected to the prostate gland and activating the nipple proceeds to influence the thymus and pancreas and eventually the pituitary gland. Men can do the breast massage techniques discussed here, but they do not get the benefit women do because they are not associated with baby milk, which contains a great deal of energy. One thing that is not different is that the kidneys store energy and control all the sexual organs. Most of the points that can be made about the breasts can be made about the testicles in a man. The method of massage is somewhat different, but they are involved with the production of orgasmic energy just as the breasts are.

Whether you are a man or a woman you have the potential to transform things into energy. You just need to know what the source of energy is. This knowledge is power that can be utilized to connect you to the universe or the Supreme Creator. You have enormous energy; in fact enough to take care of many children. Utilizing the techniques of Taoist Sexual Alchemy, you have the ability to give energy to all the vital organs in your body. Humans need to recognize that overwork, oversex, and overstimulation are bad for health. But massaging the testicles or the breasts, coupled with hand-rubbing and hand-clapping techniques, has the potential to restore and rejuvenate all the energy wasted in the foolish pursuits of overdoing things. This will cause you to feel warmth in your torso and sexual organs. You can feel the heat. As the Taoists proclaimed, it is like sun shining on the water. This process makes energy and therefore chi.

The practices discussed here, particularly those involving the sexual organs, may come into conflict with your cultural restrictions. Perhaps you are reserved about discussing some of this or perhaps you even feel it is sinful. In order to improve the quality of your life and to live you need to put this aside and adopt a more medical and energetic point of view. There is nothing sinful about love, joy, and happiness, and there certainly is not anything wrong with kindness, compassion, and helpfulness. That is what this program advocates.

SEXUAL ENERGY ACTIVATION

The first step in moving energy is to create an internal suction. For men there is a pulling sensation in the testicles and for women this is suction in the uterus. This extends up to the brain. During this process you can feel your uterus or testicles contracting and you can actually feel your brain contracting as well. Pinch gently on the nipples or massage the testicles from time to time to reactivate the energy. There should be a small amount of pain as you do this, particularly with the nipples. Concentrate on the area of your sexual organs and pull internally and the suction will commence (see fig. 5.4).

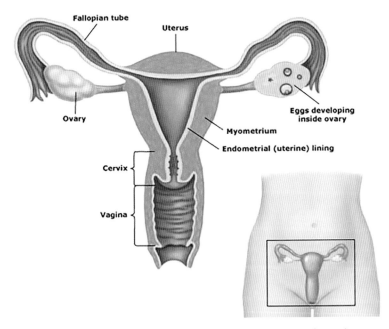

Fig. 5.4. An internal suction can be used to move energy from the uterus or testicles up to the brain.

Activate the Orgasmic Energy

1. Rub the hands together.
2. Connect to the universe so that you feel love, joy, and happiness.
3. Experience the violet light.
4. Extend your arms and hold palms of your hands toward Heaven.
5. Close your eyes.
6. Clap your hands one time.
7. Rub the hands together again to create heat.
8. Hold the breath and then relax.
9. This creates an internal suction.
10. Focus on your organs.

As you practice this exercise, the brain and the sexual organs are activated. You feel a pleasant warm sensation within you. The exercise

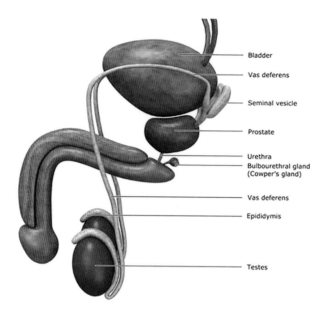

Fig. 5.5. Testicles and prostate gland are connected to the center of the brain. In women the ovaries, uterus, and vagina have a similar relationship.

is essentially the same for both men and women except for the obvious differences in the sexual organs. Women simply activate the uterus, ovaries, and vagina rather than the testicles and prostate gland. These organs have an intimate connection with the center of the brain (see fig. 5.5).

You might want to hold your nose and use your other hand to push and lift just below your navel. Focus on your uterus or prostate gland. You can actually feel the pull on the vagina, uterus, and ovaries or testicles and prostate gland. The contractions in your lower torso are accompanied by contractions in the center of the brain. The hypothalamus is activated. The more you relax the more you activate the significant organs. You will experience true happiness, which is absolutely known deep in your soul. Repetition is vital to the process. Eventually the suction will continue on its own.

The facilitator that is related to the sexual organs resides in the brain and is the hippocampus (see fig. 5.6). It is the key for con-

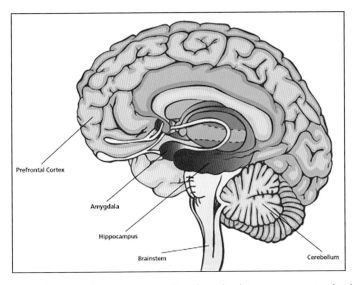

Fig. 5.6. The sexual organs are related to the hippocampus in the brain.

trolling the left and right brain as well as long-term memory. This is the way you remember the significant things about your life. It is important for you to know the location and appearance of your internal organs. Visualization is a prime mover of energy within your body.

MAKING LOVE

Many people's existence consists of constant stress with bouts of anger and other unhealthy perspectives. Unfortunately, this leads to a splitting of DNA, which results in unhealthy cells. They are a root cause of many health and psychological problems that people experience in today's world. What needs to be done is actually make love with the one person who you are truly in love with. This is a marked contrast with merely having sex. If a person just ejaculates, there is no true union. Making love involves the entire body, soul, and spirit. Union with the universal forces is not a matter of bowing, praying, or other rituals. It is a matter of love, compassion, and joy, which leads to

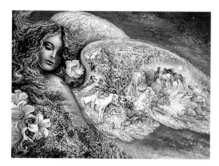

Fig. 5.7. Ambrosia is the sexual fluid of a god and goddess.

bliss. This is accessible via the proper approach to sex, which always involves love.

You can use the fantasy images of a beautiful goddess and handsome god making love. Keep in mind that when a man and woman have sex or when a god and goddess have sex they release sexual fluid. In the case of sex between a god and goddess, ambrosia or nectar is released (see fig. 5.7). You could even think of it as sacred water. When holy people have a sexual fantasy, it is a holy one, not a pornographic one. It is not something dirty or distasteful; it is good and filled with love. When you feel the god and goddess making love in your brain, your mouth will literally water as you experience the delight. Chi will enter your body from the saliva that you have generated. The energetic sexual fluid then comes down and fills the cauldron with the nectar of love. First it fills the cauldron of the throat and then it fills your entire body with love and joy. You then make love yourself to the god or goddess. When this happens you begin to feel arousal and then orgasm deep in your body throughout your brain, all the organs and glands in the body.

The same principles and approach should be true when you and the person you love have sexual intercourse. It must be approached as though it is sacred and therefore can energize and heal all the organs within you. If you do not have this attitude about it, then you are simply wasting your inner power. Your energy will be depleted. The key is to stop orgasmic outpour and replace it with Orgasmic Upward Draw as taught in the Universal Healing Tao system (see fig. 5.8).

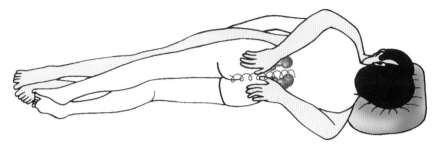

Fig. 5.8. Key to health and happiness is the Orgasmic Upward Draw, which moves the energy to the Heart point.

Simplified Upward Draw Practice

1. Upward draw of sexual energy.
2. Put the energy into all the organs.
3. Put it in the brain.
4. Facilitate a longer-lasting orgasm.
5. Improve your health and your life.
6. Become spiritually (energetically) healthier.

Breathing is an important aspect of the practice. This is simple on the one hand, but not easy to grasp initially because it involves an apparent contradiction. The essence of this is to inhale without inhaling. First you expand the lungs without inhaling. Doing this creates what can initially be thought of as an empty space. The fact is chi always fills up an empty space so that it actually is not empty. The key is mindful breathing so that you can utilize your chi properly to make your body and spirit strong. You also need to align your body with the seasons and their corresponding elements. This allows you to be rooted in Mother Earth (see fig. 5.9 on page 198).

When a person makes love according to the teachings of the Taoist masters, energy moves up to the brain instead of streaming out of the body. The orgasm is maintained within the body, which creates the brain orgasm. This is good for the brain because the cells split in a

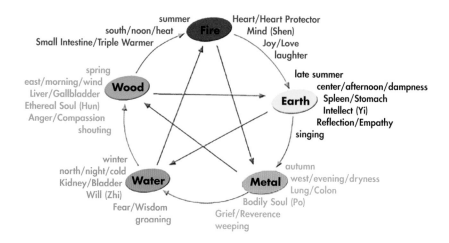

Five Elements

Generating Cycle ————▸
Control Cycle ————▸

Fig. 5.9. Tune your body to your surrounding
environment of Mother Earth, especially with the seasons.

healthy manner and facilitate the journey toward a loving and compassionate life. Such a life brings a new perspective on the world and your daily life and thus reduces negativity in the form of anger, hatred, worry, and stress.

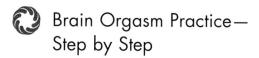 Brain Orgasm Practice—
Step by Step

1. Relax.
2. Turn your palms upward.
3. Clap.
4. Rub your hands together.
5. Massage testicles or breasts.
6. Pinch nipples.
7. Contract your prostate gland or uterus.

8. Activate diaphragm.

9. Feel arousal.

10. Move loving energy up above head.

11. Yin and yang combine.

12. Visualize god and goddess making love.

13. Brain orgasm.

14. Nectar of love fills your cauldron.

15. Overflow goes to heart and organs.

16. DNA splits.

As you make love with your partner, utilizing this process, you feel a sense of peace, joy, and love. Moreover, the DNA is repaired, renewed, and replenished. The practice is simple even though it has been held back as a mystery since ancient times.

Organ Orgasms

The culmination of this process is an organ orgasm within you. This is a long-lasting orgasm that spreads and circulates the ambrosia. A brain orgasm is capable of lasting for hours, which leads to strengthening your lungs. There are vast numbers of cells in the lungs and each one has DNA. These cells split, but the best of conditions under which they split is love, arousal, and compassion. With the proper training a lung orgasm is possible and this brings about healing and maintains healthy lungs. This practice brings the arousal and orgasm and wraps it around the lungs.

Then you can consider strengthening all of your organs. This means that you should make love without ejaculation four times a day for fifteen days. If you ejaculate you need to start over again. In this exercise, you wrap the energy around each organ. Each organ has an orgasm and produces a splitting of the DNA and therefore healthy cells result. If there is a problem with any part of the body, there is a corresponding sexual practice that can initiate repair. It can also be used as a form of maintenance in order to prevent problems. The principle in healing or maintaining the various organs is the same. The primary thing is the Orgasmic Upward Draw and wrapping the energy that has been produced around the selected part of the organ. If this is done with the positive energy of love and compassion, it produces great healing and health benefits.

Bones also need some attention in order to move along in the journey toward health and happiness. Your bones are the structure that holds you together. Bones have to be strong and this requires bone orgasms. One interesting thing about bones is that they can hold memory just like crystal can. Memories can even be passed on to the next generation through the DNA. The method for wrapping energy around the vascular system is even more lengthy and complicated, but it produces a great benefit. This is a great spiritual practice that actually rebuilds the veins and arteries. The cells split in very good condition. You need to remember that negativity brings about negativity, and thus love, joy, and happiness need to be transmitted. Of course these exercises are time consuming, but the benefits are profoundly rewarding.

BASICS OF SEXUAL MASSAGE

The ancient Taoists taught us how to transform energy and all you have to do is trust that you have fire and you were born with it. When this is combined with universal fire it can be changed to alchemical fire. There is a direct connection between the sexual organs and the brain. The Original Spirit comes from the North Star, which is the violet light. The preparation for opening up to the violet light consists of massaging the breasts or testicles. This warming process is equivalent to cooking food. It takes time to cook something properly.

Sexual massage begins with relaxing by standing up and spreading your legs: men shake their testicles loose and women shake the breasts and relax the vagina. Then accept the sacred fire and bring down the violet light to activate your orgasmic energy by raising palms upward, then clapping and rubbing the hands. After acknowledging your mid-eye

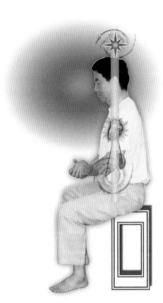

Fig. 5.10. Proper
sitting is very
important if we want
to make a connection
to positive channels.

you then massage your breasts or testicles. Following massage of the testicles or breasts, you rub the hands together again. At the same time you participate in a kind of self-confirmation and say to yourself, "I really feel it." Then you turn your palms up toward the heavens and reconnect. Sense the love, joy, and happiness of the heavens. Feel your connection to the cosmos. When you feel stress, anger, or hatred you have turned off the connection. Simply recognize that you have no connection with regard to negativity, then sit properly, smile, and relax (see fig. 5.10).

 ## Rejuvenation Procedure

The rejuvenation procedure entails sitting upright near the edge of a chair, relaxing, lifting the palms of the hands toward the heavens, and feeling the energy fill your body by expanding your awareness (see fig. 5.11 on page 202).

1. Rub your hands together in front of your face. Rub them until you begin to feel them warm up. Sometimes if you open your hands in front of your face like a book, you can actually feel the chi,

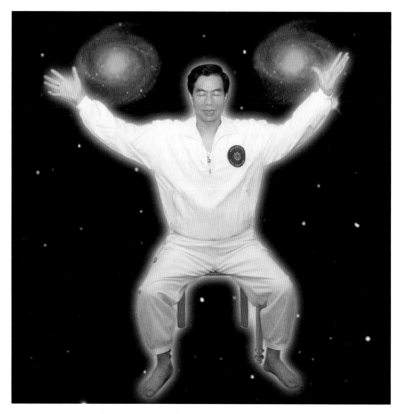

Fig. 5.11. Lift the palms of the hands toward the heavens and
feel the energy fill your body.

and at this stage you are likely able to feel as well the density of
your chi.

2. To activate the heart center, smile into it, feeling love and joy. Just
   relax and smile, relaxing your mid-eyebrow. Feel the violet light
   coming down from the North Star to your crown and your uplifted
   palms. Smile, relax, and feel love, joy, and happiness. Relax your
   mid-eyebrow and crown and the violet light will come to you.

3. Slowly the violet light will get darker and thicker. You feel joy as
   your palms absorb the violet light from the North Star. Taoists
   believe that this fire can transform everything. Hold your hands
   with palms up toward the heaven and feel the fire.

Basic Breast and Testicle Massage

1. Stand and bounce, shaking your breasts or testicles, then sit with hands up and out at shoulder level drawing in Primordial Force.

2. **Women:** Warm your hands and massage your breasts with your palms on your nipples inwardly (24–36 times). Rest and hold breasts (see fig. 5.12).

   Men: Sit up and warm hands, cupping and warming testicles, then massage testicles and scrotum drawing sexual energy into kidneys to warm them. Rest and hold testicles.

3. **Both:** Repeat and feel the heat.

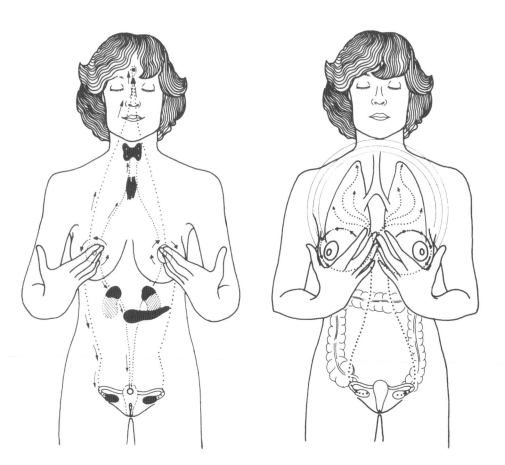

Fig. 5.12. Breast massage

4. **Women:** Massage breasts outwardly, drawing energy into all the vital organs and glands.

  Men: Massage testicles again, drawing energy to kidneys and brain.
5. Rest, hold, and feel the energy.

Take time to massage yourself. Be patient and relax as you do it. When doing this, it must be done properly and patiently because it is a process. Transformation consumes time; this is a fact of life. In men, the testicle massage, following the appropriate amount of time, sends the energy from the testicles to the kidneys then to the brain itself. This revitalizes the brain. The energy that is produced in this procedure is more powerful than sexual energy because it is the multiplication of sexual energy hundreds and thousands of times.

ACTIVATION, TRANSFORMATION, AND CONSERVATION OF ENERGY IN THE BODY

Transformation has several meanings and different people understand it in different ways. Having a meaningful and deep comprehension of transformation is vital in the practice of Taoism. It is something that you need to understand because it relates to the importance of orbits and the organs. The conservation of energy is assisted, in the case of human beings, because humans are the only creatures capable of producing energy. Witness the simple act of starting a fire. No other animal can do that. Science tells us that conservation of energy coupled with finding alternative sources of energy is vital in the modern world.

You need to focus on having a meaningful relationship with everything you do. You cannot have your mind one way, your eyes another way, and your hands another way. That causes the spirit and soul to be scattered in relation to energy. One result of this is that you do not get anything accomplished. The Taoist approach is threefold: focus, concentrate, and conserve energy. The mid-eye, bridge of the nose, and tip of the nose link the mind, heart, spirit, and soul together. Awareness of this link helps prevent you from becoming too scattered (see fig. 5.13).

The foundational practices of Sexual Alchemy involve activation, linking, and focusing. Done properly, they result in a sharper and clearer focus and centering of your energy. The ordinary mind comes together with the logical mind, opening up more of your brain. This is significant because science has shown us that people only use a fraction of their brain. Radar is a good analogy to understand these principles. The radar is like conscious awareness. Suppose you had a very good radar system and a very good monitor. The most important thing is that someone is watching the monitor. The people watching the monitor have to have the knowledge, wisdom, and understanding of what is being picked up.

These basic learning processes are actually training your spirit and soul. The spirit and soul never sleep and are aware of many things you do not have in your conscious mind. The spirit and soul are filled with

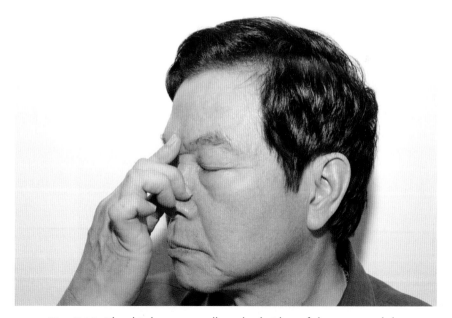

Fig. 5.13. The third eye as well as the bridge of the nose and the tip of the nose are important for proper focus.

useful knowledge, but they are unable to communicate it to your consciousness. It is almost as though the spirit and soul and your awareness speak different languages. To put it another way, your spirit and soul are always present and always there, but you do not realize everything that is happening. To realize the totality of your experience you need to turn inward. This permits you to expand outward and become a more awakened person. Enlightenment is a matter of being awake and nothing more. A simple formula for this is "consciousness in and awareness out."

To understand the Tao you must include understanding the violet light. We know from numerous photos that the universe looks like the human brain. The spirit and soul are intelligent energy. The violet light, along with all the connections it makes, has intelligence (see fig. 5.14).

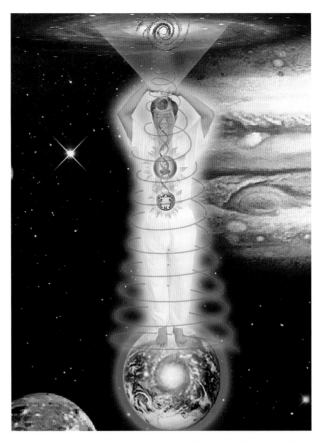

Fig. 5.14. Violet light connects to the brain and has intelligence.

The pulsing of the North Star, which influences the earth's pulse, also affects your heart pulse, the pulse in your kidneys, and the pulse in other organs. The pulse of the North Star, precisely because it causes the heart to pump, is responsible for life. If you ask the North Star for life, if you connect to it, and if you have faith in it, your life will be healthy and happy for a long time. Simply attach your being to the inexhaustible pulse of the North Star.

You need to recognize and utilize the force of the violet light, the highest form of light in the universe. Open your mid-eye to experience it and recognize the infinite power of love available in every corner of the cosmos. Trust that love, joy, and happiness are stored in the heart. Always remember the Inner Smile, which draws the violet light. This process ignites a loving fire. With sufficient practice and patience you will be able to kindle the alchemical fire.

Awaken the Fire Dragon

Many of the problems of the world could be solved if there were a basic understanding of how our structure works and what it does. There are problems associated with being bipeds who walk upright. This is one reason why the area of the coccyx is so important. Many nerves end near the coccyx, so every time it is activated, the result goes all the way up to the brain. In addition, this is also where the sacral pump is located. When this pump does not work, the brain is unable to work properly, because it is not receiving enough spinal fluid. Animals do not have this problem, but people do because we are bipeds who walk erect. The way to deal with such problems is to get your coccyx moving. That will awaken the sleeping dragon and transform it into a swimming dragon that swims upward. It goes all the way up and connects to the forces in the heavens (see fig. 5.15 on page 208).

You begin with imagining your tail extending downward to the ground. The key is to make sure your coccyx is totally relaxed and loose. As you relax downward, your body will be activated by the energy

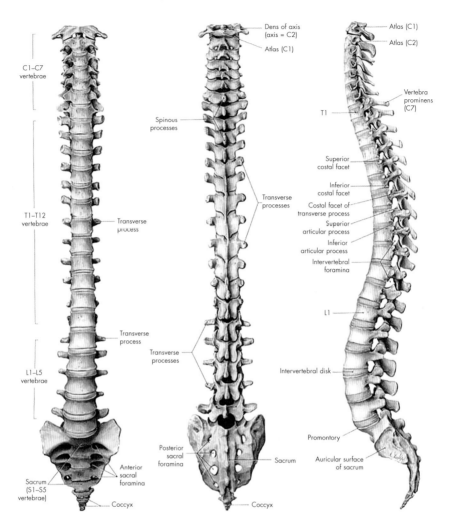

Fig. 5.15. The human spine: vertebrae, sacrum, and coccyx

from Mother Earth. A vibration will commence. This vibration is like a dragon tail. Relax even more and the Fire Dragon will begin to warm your coccyx. You will feel the energy moving upward. The heat will spread to your kidneys and other organs. It then will extend upward to the brain itself. As the activated Fire Dragon streams upward, the North Star, Big Dipper, and violet light come down. At the same time the Dragon's Tail extends deep into Mother Earth.

Activation of Coccyx and Sacrum Practice

1. Relax—up, down, and in.
2. Stand up.
3. Rub your tailbone (coccyx).
4. Rub your sacrum.
5. Tap the back of your skull and your eyes will roll upward. Be sure to smile and hold on to the image of the North Star and the Big Dipper.
6. Relax, let go, and feel the upward pulling force of the North Star.

The practice utilized in activating the sacral pump mimics an erotic dance. Standing up, you move the pelvis forward and back, almost as in sexual intercourse. Then do this in reverse, extending the buttocks outward and back. Finally move side to side. This gets the pump pushing upward and reverses the flow of downward energy (or the loss of energy). The energy goes up to the crown, connecting to the infinite cosmic forces, which will infuse you with additional energy.

Opening the Door of Life

The Door of Life on the spine, like all doors, opens and closes (see fig. 5.16 on page 210). You need to really feel the spine opening and closing. This is quite significant because it relates to the health of your organs, including the kidneys. To open the Door of Life, you stand up, bend the knees a little, and lean forward slightly. As you inhale and expand the chest, an alchemical fire will be ignited, which will then move to the chest. Then you exhale and curve the chest inward.

You also need to take care of your neck by bending your head forward so the chin touches the chest. This means that the crown toward the back portion of the top of your head points toward the North Star. Put another way, you can think of the crown as a mountain. When your head is moved forward, the mountain points directly to the heavens. This is important if you want to make a connection. As the crown

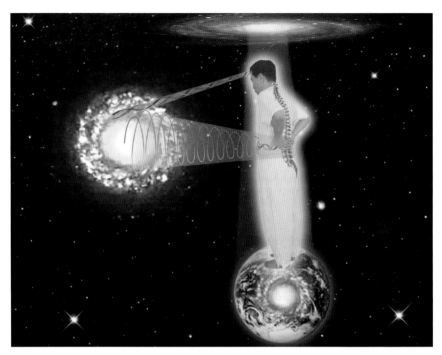

Fig. 5.16. Opening the Door of Life has a positive influence
on your organs and overall health.

points upward, the force will enter and go right down the spine. You can
clasp your hands behind your head to help you push your chin down to
your chest. Pull your elbows together to move your head forward.

During this exercise you must make sure you are properly grounded.
You need the support of Mother Earth. This simply means that you
need to have the proper stance. Your feet must be planted firmly on the
ground about shoulder-width apart. Your toes should be pointed straight
ahead. Bend the knees slightly a few times to confirm your stance.

Open the Door of Life (Abbreviated)

1. Inhale with arms upward, shoulders back, and chest expanded.
2. Exhale, arms in front, pointed up with fists clenched, shoulders forward, chest curved inward, and back rounded.

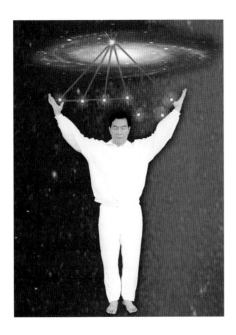

Fig. 5.17. Tucking the chin aligns the crown of the head with the North Star.

3. Bend your head forward so the chin touches the chest. This will align the crown of your head with the North Star (see fig. 5.17). Use your index finger to push the chin to the chest and then release. Repeat.
4. Rub your hands together and feel energy moving up and down your spine. Feel your pumps pumping as the spinal fluid moves up and down.
5. Sit down and rock your spine.

When you have completed this exercise properly you will receive a blessing from the heavens.

The Gate of Life and Death

The Hui Yin (perineum region) is called the Gate of Life and Death. If sexual energy leaks out, organ energy leaks out, and the result is death. It is up to you to open the Gate of Life and not the Gate of Death. The connection that your Hui Yin point makes runs up the spine and continues all the way up to your brain. It is a crossroads. The front connects to the sexual organs and the back connects to the anus. The sexual organs control your sexual energy and the anus controls the energy in your organs. The lower link connects to the soles of the feet, which are placed on Mother Earth. The earth is yin and that energy courses up to the sexual organs. Getting in touch with yourself and especially your organs is of great importance. The energy of your sexual organs can be replenished if you do the necessary sexual exercises.

As you move your focus to the Hui Yin, hold it and massage it a little. Apply pressure firmly as you might do in a massage. Press, contract, and then hold the Hui Yin as you hold your breath. Energy will start to gather in the region. Feel yourself gather sexual energy, earth energy, and organ energy. This is like a well that gathers water, and the deeper and wider you dig the more it can store. Practice in silence, then smile and relax while the focus returns to the Hui Yin.

You can work on your Hui Yin each day. It will open more and more, and this facilitates the ability to collect more energy. This is a longevity practice. It rejuvenates and refreshes the body and helps you have a longer and healthier life. You can do this exercise standing or sitting.

Gate of Life and Death (Hui Yin) Practice

1. Use the finger and touch the Hui Yin.
2. Inhale.
3. Press.
4. Exhale.
5. Focus.
6. Hold your breath.
7. Smile.
8. Rock just a little.
9. Continue rocking and relaxing into your Hui Yin.
10. Activate the channel running from the Hui Yin to the anus, which you must contract, to the coccyx, and up to the middle of the back.

Run the energy up this channel 9 times. Hold after the ninth time. You may use your finger to hold it if you prefer.

You need to do this at least 36 times. With practice, you will not need to use your finger. You will feel the energy move into your sexual organs (testicles for men and uterus and ovaries for women). When your sexual organs are properly activated you will see the violet light; that is an indication that the sexual energy is transforming.

Rocking aids in holding the breath much longer. As you relax and exhale, every time you breathe in, you will feel the energizing breath go deep into your being. As the ancient Taoists say, the breath strives to dive deep into the sea. The Hui Yin exercises are the beginning of the practice of alchemy. Just as oil is added to a lamp to make a bright light shine, each time you breathe in, it is like you are gathering oil and water. As you inhale and pull into the coccyx, you pump the oil into the tan tien fire. When the preparation is done, the soles of your feet and the crown of your head are activated. You have more life added to your being so that you can finish your work and assure that the time spent here has meaning. You are, in essence, feeding your soul and spirit.

Make sure to breathe as you feel the prostate gland, testicles, and scrotum or uterus, ovaries, and vagina. The prostate gland/uterus as well as the anus are breathing. Inhale and exhale as you feel the smiling sunshine enter your body and spirit. Nice warm energy will enter your body. Then you want to move the energy to the Hua Hin, the area in the lower abdomen where the four yin yang symbols spin (see fig. 2.22 on page 75). The spinning of the four chi balls produces more chi.

Add Fire to the Kidneys

There is kidney fire and tan tien fire. You must keep these fires burning or the lamp will burn out. Your brain has nerves that connect to your kidneys. The heart provides these vital organs with the life force

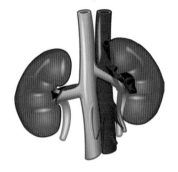

Fig. 5.18. Kidneys are vital
to health and happiness.

of blood. See your kidneys and know them (fig. 5.18). Look into them
with your inner eye.

As you are visualizing and caring for your kidneys, do the following simple breathing exercise to activate and improve the kidney pulse.
Oxygen and carbon dioxide are balancing as your kidneys get warmer.
As you hold your breath, suction commences in the abdomen. Your testicles or ovaries and kidneys breathe.

Kidney Activation

1. Warm palms, close your eyes, waving them left and right.
2. Cup kidneys, inhale; hold breath for 30–60 seconds until you have
   suction.
3. Exhale; hold your breath until you feel suction.
4. Then relax and breathe normally. Rest and collect the energy.
5. With eyes closed, roll eyes down, back, up, and front, and reverse,
   with a slow breath activating the olfactory nerve (see fig. 5.19).

The olfactory nerve has a connection to the thalamus, hypothalamus, and pituitary glands. The olfactory bulb connects the hypothalamus to all the other glands. Normal and shallow breathing will not
stimulate the olfactory nerve. Small and long sip breathing will stimulate the olfactory bulb and thereby all the other glands. Replenishing
your kidney helps to open the Gate of Life and avoid the Gate of
Death.

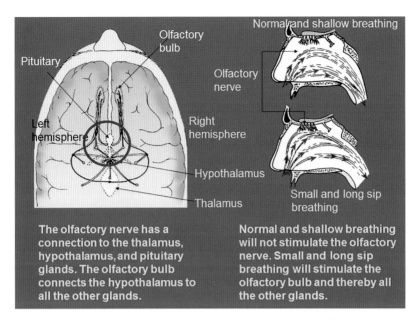

Fig. 5.19. Use the olfactory nerve and breathe into the eyes.

Add Fire to the Tan Tien

When the fire is activated in your kidneys and lower tan tien, chi will ascend to the brain. You will be connected to the earth and the universe. As you gather Earth Chi, you need to smile and be aware of the galaxy. You should connect to the boundless energy of the sun and moon (see fig. 5.20 on page 216). While this natural process is taking place, concentrate on your sexual organs to initiate the flow of energy and then gather chi into your lower tan tien.

Trust that you have a bio-battery that is rechargeable. Note that this takes place during a sound and motionless sleep. During your waking hours, you can focus and relax while drawing in the cosmic energy of the North Star and violet light. Rub your stomach and charge the intestines. Do not be embarrassed if this causes you to expel gas. Invite the chi to be with you.

The chi that you acquire should be stored in the abdomen because the brain and the heart are too hot for it (see fig. 5.21 on page 216).

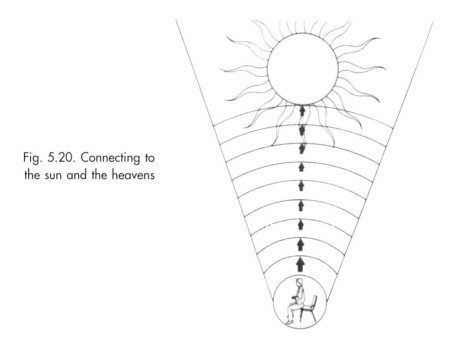

Fig. 5.20. Connecting to the sun and the heavens

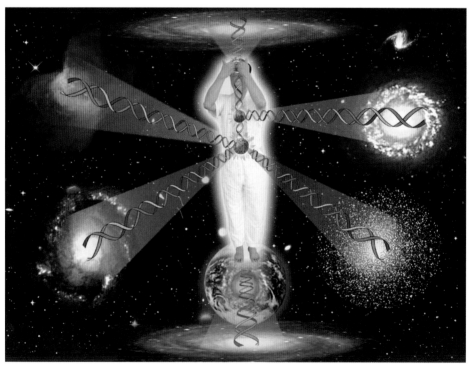

Fig. 5.21. Condense the chi in your abdominal tan tien.

Grasping the principle of storing chi in your abdominal chi ball is essential to the practice of Taoism. Remember to trust, invite, and then store. Visualize and align yourself correctly and you are on your way to enlightenment.

There are many roads to enlightenment. There is chi everywhere, there is godhead everywhere, the force is everywhere, and there are pulses everywhere. The forces that impact you come from the north, south, east, and west, which results in an orbit. Such an orbit is essentially infinite, so holding on to the orbit and going with it means immortality. Always bear in mind that you also have the Microcosmic Orbit. It too has no beginning and no end and is a tool for joining together with the eternal and infinite orbit of the cosmos itself. Everything finds a balance and has equal power. Numerous illustrations whose origins date back hundreds of years indicate many of the points along the spine. The ancient pictures often show a water buffalo pulling a water cart up the human spine. Below is a modern way of making the same point (see fig. 5.22).

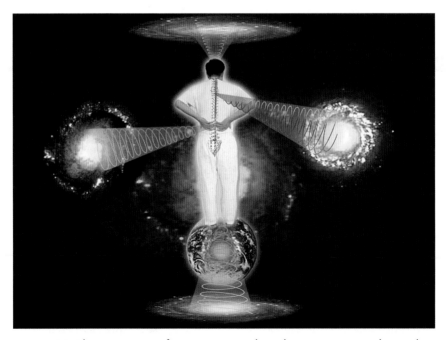

Fig. 5.22. The movement of energy pumped up the spine is critical in order to establish a polarity with the North Star and Southern Cross.

The lower tan tien is the primary energy reserve in your body. You store the energy you generate in that area. You can replenish this energy through the chi ball, which spins along with the four Tai Chi symbols. Because energy dissipates, it is important that you connect with both Mother Earth and the galaxy, bringing cosmic energy back down through your crown, down the spine, and into your kidneys. Your lower tan tien restores and replenishes your kidney fire. You can access the energy-condensing region of the navel as you exhale during your practice. You will find yourself worrying less and not thinking too much. While the energy is in the area of your navel, it is important to keep the throat clear. You want to allow the free flow of energy to move down your spine. You are actually connected to the universe. Your body and mind are recharged through deep breathing and letting go. Science agrees in verifying these connections more and more.

Lower Tan Tien Exercise

1. Open the crown and activate the pineal gland.
2. Move the energy down through your throat.
3. Move energy down to the heart.
4. Move it down to the solar plexus.
5. Move it back down to the navel.
6. Orbit and inhale.
7. Contract the Hui Yin (perineum region) and anus.
8. Slowly look upward and concentrate on your spine.
9. Look up to the crown and hold for a moment.
10. Open your mid-eye and hold.
11. Reach down to the tip of the tongue and palate.
12. Exhale.
13. Move energy back to Hui Yin and contract.
14. Move it to the coccyx and sacrum.
15. Inhale and exhale down.

16. Breathe—inhale and exhale with a conscious mind.

17. Repeat.

Ask the chi to be with you as you condense and store the energy. You are surrounded by energetic orbits, all of which have an impact on you. From the smallest electron to the stars and planets, you can connect with these sources of energy. The more you spin your orbits, the more energy will be provided to you. All you need to do is understand the cyclical nature of the universe and flow with it. That is the Way of the Tao. Nature abounds with energy. Do not waste your energy with negative emotions or stressful situations. Remember you can recycle it to Mother Earth and she transforms it into positive energy back to you.

SPIRITUAL LOVE

At this point in your practice you can visualize a god and goddess making love. An amazing aesthetic experience takes place as you stimulate your being into an arousal, which eventually results in the spilling of ambrosia and elixir into the cauldron in your brain. The power of this elixir of life spreads throughout your body until you yourself are making love with the Divine. You become united with the universe as yin and yang come together and form the Eternal Tao. You now have the ability to connect into this infinite chi and refill your existence with love, joy, and happiness. Add life into your life.

There are stories and sacred texts describing this in traditions from around the world. For all, the ambrosia is seen as the nectar of life. These texts show how highly the sacred cauldron is ranked in traditions from both the East and West. For all these traditions, there is an element of the sacred that connects us to the Divine (violet light). Your cauldrons of nectar are heated up with the internal fires of your being. You reach a loving and compassionate orgasm, which spreads through your body; negativity dissipates and the violet light replaces it. This cycle continues and you remain connected to the cosmic power or the original force.

This is a state of spiritual love and sex. The physical unification enables the spiritual and universal unification to activate as you give and receive love, joy, and happiness. To transition to a more sexual state for beginning Sexual Alchemy, you might want to lie down and relax your sexual organs.

Preparation for Sexual Alchemy

1. Peacefully and quietly lie down. Give your body permission to get aroused sexually. Smile to your sexual organs and open yourself to the violet light. Remember that visualization is conducive to sexual arousal and orgasm. Let your inhibitions go and experience the bliss and joy of energizing chi.

2. While you are reclining, stretch the lumbar and sacrum. Hold your knees with your arms and locked hands. Pull them toward the chest. Feel your lumbar open (see fig. 5.23).

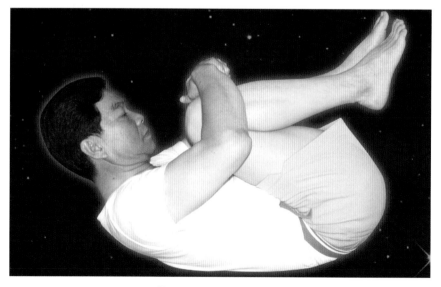

Fig. 5.23. Pull your knees up toward your chest.

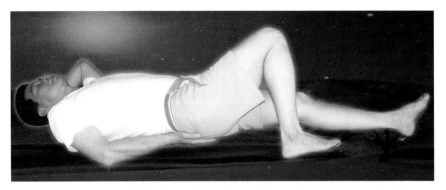

Fig. 5.24. Stretch the knee of one leg while reclining on your back.

3. Then cross one leg over the other while lying on your back. Push your knee down toward the floor (see fig. 5.24).
4. Then do the other leg. If your body is relaxed and open, then your spirit and soul will be as well.

There are numerous stretching exercises that can open your spine and other parts of your body to prepare for the erotic dance of love leading to orgasm. You can discover what works for you, but the lumbar and sacrum generally need to be open. This facilitates the flow of erotic nectar from the gods. Being armored in any aspect of your body or spirit is counterproductive and creates a barrier to the joining of two beings. Every aspect of your body, spirit, and soul needs to be open.

Stretching Exercise

Sitting on the floor and grasping your toes is one of the most important stretches (see fig. 5.25 on page 222). Make sure to keep your head up as you do this. If you are not quite able to grasp your toes, use a towel. This should be done daily with a lot of repetitions, perhaps as many as seventy. You can say "do not leave home without it" as a memory device so that you are sure to stretch before you undertake your daily activities.

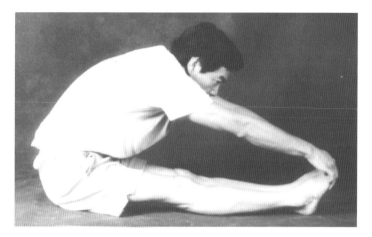

Fig. 5.25. Sit on the floor with legs flat and grasp your toes with head up.

1. Sit on the floor.
2. Stretch, grasping your toes with head up.
3. Rest.
4. Guide chi into tendons and ligaments.
5. Chi flows into spine and organs.

This approach to the practice was passed on to ancient China from India. The Chinese added their own techniques, with many aspects of the martial arts and kung fu. The Chinese approach to meditation was also added in some schools. A very strong emphasis on the tendons was a significant part of ancient Taoism. The martial arts, however, did not emphasize exercises done lying down but did highlight the lumbar and the hips. The main point is to be supple and loose and the tendons are critical in this regard.

SINGLE CULTIVATION PRACTICES

Cultivating, conserving, redirecting, and circulating the generative force from the sexual organs to higher centers of the body invigorates and rejuvenates all the vital functions and activates the higher forces.

Male Sexual Alchemy

Although the principle of conservation applies to both men and women, the actual practice of conserving Ching Chi differs. In studying the nature of sex, Taoist masters found that the main way men lose Ching Chi is through ejaculation. They developed a way to control and use sexual energy through the practices of Testicle Breathing, Scrotal Compression, Genital Massage, Power Lock, the Orgasmic Upward Draw, and others. By learning to separate orgasm and ejaculation—two distinct physical processes—men can transform a momentary release into countless peaks of whole body orgasms without losing an erection. In addition to becoming better sexual partners, multi-orgasmic men enjoy increased vitality and longevity because they minimize the fatigue and depletion that follow ejaculation.

Female Sexual Alchemy

Women lose little sexual energy through orgasm, but instead lose it primarily through menstruation and childbearing. The sexual guidance and exercises of the Universal Healing Tao system are being introduced plainly to the Western public for the first time. For thousands of years Taoist masters taught these secrets only to very small numbers of people in the royal courts and in esoteric circles, who were sworn to silence. There are three main practices that women can use to cultivate and enhance their sexual energy: Ovarian Breathing and Compression, Breast Massage, the Orgasmic Upward Draw, and Chi Weight Lifting. When these practices are mastered one can experience a total body orgasm that is beyond ordinary vaginal orgasm. A series of exercises with a jade or stone egg are used to strengthen the urogenital and pelvic diaphragm, the muscles of the vagina, and the glands, tendons, and nervous system. These practices can shorten menstruation, reduce cramps, and compress more life-force energy (chi) into the ovaries for more sexual and creative power. These exercises lend themselves to titters by the uninformed, but in fact they have been successfully practiced for thousands of years to enhance the potency and pleasure of the women fortunate enough to know about them.

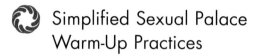 Simplified Sexual Palace Warm-Up Practices

The Sexual Palace is located at the pubic bone for both men and women; in women it is named the Ovarian Palace and in men the Sperm Palace.

1. Warm palms and massage kidneys (18 times). Rest; then do 3 more sets.
2. Warm hands and massage testicles/ovaries (9 times). Rest; then do 3 more sets.
3. **Men:** Hold testicles with left palm. Right palm massage abdomen to navel clockwise (36–81 times). Rest. Reverse.
   Women: Massage ovaries with warm hands down to vagina and back (36–81 times).
4. Gather chi ball in navel and Door of Life, then condense them. Draw lower tan tien into one chi ball.
5. Cover sexual area; use mind power to connect with iris muscle (the muscle controlling the constriction of the pupil in the eye), Gate of Life and Death, and anus, then contract them.
6. Expand all of the areas as you exhale into tan tien.

Simplified Male Sexual Chi Massage

1. Internal Belly Breathing: Place middle fingers 1.5 inches below navel and inhale into fingers, then exhale, releasing breath (81 times).
2. Kidney Warmer: Stand and warm hands, then place on kidneys, bending forward slightly as you inhale, pulling up anus to kidneys. Exhale, deflating and warming kidneys, drawing energy up (36 times).

3. Power Lock: Inhale (small sips) into the crown (3 times).

4. Massage genitals, perineum, and sacrum with a silk cloth and spiral 36 times (first clockwise and then counterclockwise), with testicles loose and full of chi.

5. Testicle Finger Massage: Hold testicles with right and left hands then press thumbs on testicles and massage them 36 times (first clockwise and then counterclockwise). Roll them left, right, back, and up 36 times (see fig. 5.26).

6. Testicle Palm Massage: Hold testicles with left palm, lightly press, then rub gently with left palm 36 times, first clockwise and then counterclockwise. Warm hands and do reverse, drawing energy up to crown.

7. Ducts Elongation Rub: Cup testicles, then trace ducts up and down using thumbs and index fingers, drawing energy to crown.

8. Ducts Stretching Massage: Hold ducts with right thumb and rub

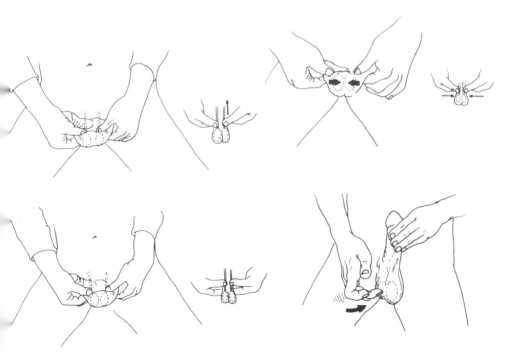

Fig. 5.26. In the Taoist practice massaging the testicles is very important.

with index finger. Gently pull testicles out, stretching ducts, and massage testicles. Repeat 36 times, drawing energy up.

9. Scrotum and Penis Tendons' Stretch: Encircle base of penis with thumb and index finger, then pull entire groin down and pull internal organs up, left and right. Hold, then release, drawing energy up to crown (36 times clockwise and then 36 times counterclockwise).

10. Penis Massage: Use thumbs and index fingers to hold penis base; draw energy up, then massage penis along left, right, and middle lines from base to tip (36 times).

11. Testicle Tapping: Inhale, pulling up, holding breath, clenching teeth, contracting perineum and anus. Lift penis with left fingers, lightly tap right testicle (9 times), then exhale and rest, drawing energy up spine to crown (reverse to left testicle).

Simplified Female Sexual Chi Massage

1. Internal Belly Breathing: Place middle fingers 1.5 inches below navel and inhale into fingers, then exhale, releasing breath (81 times).

2. Kidney Warmer: Stand and warm hands, then place on kidneys, bending forward slightly, and inhale, pulling up anus to kidneys. Exhale, deflating and warming kidneys, drawing energy up (36 times).

3. Power Lock: Inhale (small sips) into the crown (3 times).

4. Massage perineum, sacrum, and vaginal muscles: Press on groin with silk cloth over three fingers, spiraling 36 times to activate the chi. Start to feel breasts enlarge and vagina moistening.

5. Breast Massage: Get in seated position, with pressure against vagina (by sitting up against a hard object, or placing a rolled up towel between your legs). Pull up anus, drawing chi up through spine. Pull up left and right anus, bringing chi up to nipples. Warm hands, place tongue on palate, and place the second joint of the middle finger of each hand directly on the nipple

of its respective breast. Cup the outside of the breasts with your palms.

6. Gland Massage: Place the three middle fingers on each breast, then circle outward from nipples, then inward, drawing chi from energized clitoris to the head, activating pineal, pituitary, thyroid, thymus, pancreas, and adrenal glands, accumulating chi back at breasts.

7. Organ Massage: Warm hands, cover and circle breasts, feeling chi from thymus and activating lungs accumulate at breasts, then direct to heart, spleen, kidneys, and liver. Cover pelvic area, feeling chi expand into nipples and down to ovaries. Feel pulsation of vagina (opening and closing) drawing chi to Ovarian Palace. Squeeze cervix, hold, relax, and absorb chi.

8. Ovaries Massage: Place hands on ovaries and massage with silk cloth 36 times in both directions, stimulating breasts and clitoris (vaginal secretions will signal readiness for egg insertion—see Egg Exercise below).

Simplified Testicle and Ovarian Breathing

1. Standing or sitting: Scrotum hanging free or focus on ovaries with tongue to palate, palms on knees, chin tucked in, head high, eyes closed, smile down and do Microcosmic Orbit (3 times).

2. Lying down on right side, pillow raising head, right fingers in front of right ear, right thumb sits behind right ear, left hand on left thigh, right leg straight and left leg bent.

3. Be aware of testicles or ovaries spiraling to feel sexual energy, then inhale slowly through nose, pulling genitals up, hold, exhale slowly, lower genitals, feel cool energy in scrotum or vagina, then inhale up to Sexual Palace (9 counts each time), up to perineum, sacrum, kidneys, T11, point opposite heart, C7, Jade Pillow, and crown. Then exhale, spiraling into brain (36 times) feeling a little blissfulness (see fig. 5.27 on page 228).

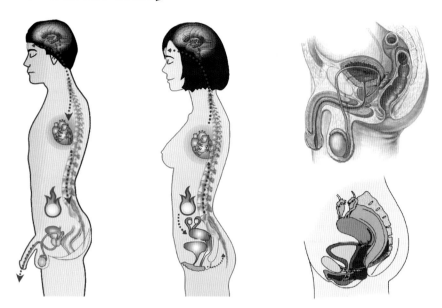

Fig. 5.27. Testicle and Ovarian Breathing and
Scrotal and Ovarian Compression

Simplified Scrotal and Ovarian Compression

1. Do Testicle or Ovarian Breathing sitting, inhaling through nose.
2. Swallow air (imaginary energy ball), pushing down to solar plexus, navel, abdomen, and scrotum or vagina.
3. Forcefully compress air into scrotum or vagina, swallowing air again; hold breath 30–60 seconds while squeezing anal and perineal muscles, then exhale. Swallow saliva and relax tongue to palate.
4. Rest and repeat with bellows breathing to start (93 times).
5. Collect energy at navel. Do Bone Breathing.

Simplified Power Lock (Orgasmic Upward Draw)

1. Sitting or standing, stimulate Jade Staff (penis) or vagina to 90 percent of orgasmic erection or wetness. Use mind to arouse penis or vagina by spiraling at the gland and concentrate.

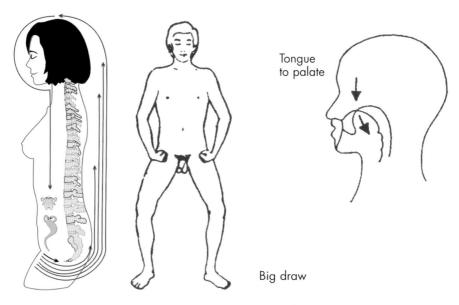

Tongue
to palate

Big draw

Fig. 5.28. Orgasmic Upward Draw

2. Inhale with clawed feet, clenched fists and buttocks, tucked-in chin, clenched teeth, tongue to palate; pull in eyes and look up to crown, closing eyes and using the mind (see fig. 5.28).

3. Hold, then inhale again, drawing up energy to genitals and anus region; pull energy to perineum by lightly squeezing.

4. Hold to 9 counts (muscles fully flexed, which means lightly contracted), then exhale, releasing all muscles in the body. Be aware of orgasm energy rising up, then do Microcosmic Orbit.

5. Follow same procedure, then draw up to sacrum, to T11, C7, and Jade Pillow (C1), then up to crown. Rest. Use mind power to guide orgasm feeling up to crown (see fig. 5.29 on page 230).

6. Practice draw until erection or wetness subsides (6 contractions) with sexual energy travelling from penis or vagina to crown in Governor Channel, going from station to station.

7. When sexual energy fills crown, spiral (36 times), feel connection with universe (blissful feeling). Bring it down to the mid-eyebrow, nose, palate, tongue, throat, heart, solar plexus, and navel.

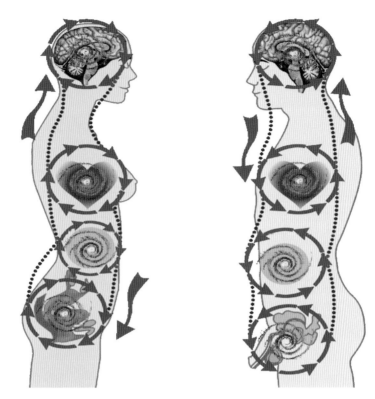

Fig. 5.29. Draw orgasm energy up the spine.

8. Exhale, relaxing whole body. Cover your navel with both palms (left over right for men, right over left for women). Collect and mentally spiral the energy outwardly from the navel 36 times (clockwise for men, counterclockwise for women) and then inwardly 24 times (counterclockwise for men, clockwise for women)

Simplified Female Egg Exercise

1. In Horse stance (feet shoulder-width apart and firmly grounded, ankles and knees bent, groin folded, spine and neck in alignment), insert jade egg into vagina with large end first (use lubricant), then contract muscles to close external vaginal orifice tightly, keeping egg in vaginal canal (see fig. 5.30).

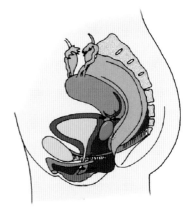

Fig. 5.30. Female Egg Exercise

2. Inhale while contracting vaginal canal muscles in front of cervix (contracting two sections at same time).
3. Slightly squeeze egg (good grip), then inhale, squeezing gradually; finally inhale further, squeezing harder and slowly moving egg up and down, increasing to faster motion, then exhale.
4. Move egg left and right using top and bottom of vaginal canal muscles.
5. Tilt egg up and down, top and bottom, moving it up to touch cervix, then down to external orifice, then release.

MULTI-ORGASMIC COUPLE

Men and women have different sexual energies—and too often this leads to disharmony, preventing us from fully exploring our sexual potential. By harnessing the power of an ancient tradition of sexual wisdom you and your partner can learn to use physical and psychological techniques to experience the bliss of a whole body sexual experience with orgasm after orgasm. The unique "sexercises" presented here can help anyone go deeper into a loving relationship. The art that has evolved over centuries of Taoist understanding can be brought to life again today to further expand the healing power for lovers. Couples will find and increase their sexual energy potential and deepen their

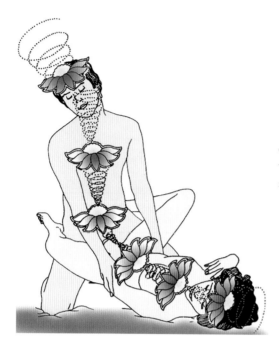

Fig. 5.31. The sexual energy is sent upward to the brain, which then spirals in the brain.

physical compatibility, as well as develop an ecstatic form of acupressure. This is sexuality taught as a way for health and healing, spiritual growth, and longevity.

The theory of Healing Love is chicken soup. What is chicken soup? You take a chicken and put it in a pot of water and boil it for two hours, then take the chicken out. Which would you rather eat, the chicken or the broth? The broth is what you would eat because the broth has all the essence of the chicken in it, while the chicken meat would taste like rubber. Try it. The chicken is your genitals and you cook them with the Universal Healing Tao Healing Love practices, then draw their essence out of them and up your spine into your brain (see fig. 5.31). Instead of a genital orgasm (outside the body in men) you will experience a total body orgasm (because the brain is connected to all the parts of your body). You lose none of your sexual fluids (semen and hormones), which you need daily to create every cell of the body. These same formulas apply to women for the loss of sexual fluids during their menstrual cycle.

You have the ability to completely experience your sexual energy and take it to new highs without losing any of your vital creative energy. You achieve this by cultivating it through the Healing Love practices to heal yourself and your loved one. Through these practices you will learn and experience the ability to manage your sexual energy instead of it controlling you. In Dual Cultivation you start to understand through the practices of the Orgasmic Upward Draw, total body orgasm, and the Valley Orgasm (Shallow and Thrusting techniques). You will learn how to work together with your partner to heal yourselves and flow together in a harmonious, monogamous, long-lasting relationship.

Anatomical Insights

There are obvious differences between men and women, but it should be noted that at conception there are essentially no differences. The differences develop over time (see fig. 5.32 on page 234). Eventually the penis develops as well as the clitoris.

In an adult male the penis is big when compared to the clitoris of an adult female. The entry to the vagina is, relatively speaking, some distance from the clitoris. In spite of the apparent relative smallness of the clitoris, it is quite big because what is seen is essentially like the tip of the iceberg. In the frontal portion of the vagina the labia minor come together and make a fold of skin termed the prepuce. The clitoris is located under the prepuce. The clitoris is a structure of roughly three fourths of an inch of highly sensitive tissue that swells with blood when sexually stimulated. Below the vaginal opening are the labia minor which meet at the fourchette and behind the fourchette is the anus. Between the vagina and the anus is the perineum.

Women are water oriented, which means that fluid is necessary. There are glands that produce the female sexual fluids, which are different fluids than come from a man. They are of major importance for sexual intercourse. In Taoist terms, you cannot sail your boat in a dry

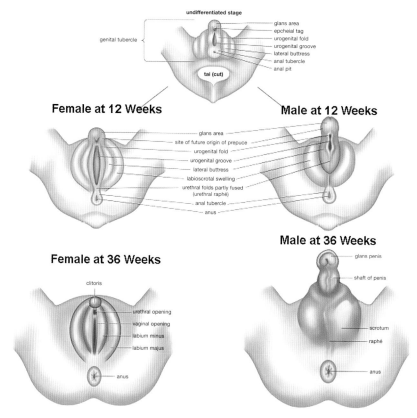

Fig. 5.32. Initially there is no difference between a
male fetus and a female fetus.

river. Meaningful sexual intercourse necessitates the man being patient and compassionate. While a woman is water, a man is fire. He needs to have enough fire to heat up the water in the female.

With the interconnections of all aspects of the body, many organs are involved in the process of making love. Among those are the sexual organs, the bladder, the prostate gland, the uterus, and the vagina. Many women become aware of this interconnection of the organs and even men have some concept of it because of what the ancient Taoists call the Mysterious Gate. In the West, this has become known as the G-spot (see fig. 5.33). The term G-spot is named for the German gynecologist Ernst Gräfenberg. It is an erogenous area in the vagina that, when properly stimulated, leads to strong sexual arousal and profound orgasms. It is located 2–3 inches in front of the vaginal wall and between the vaginal opening and the urethra. Sometimes when activated, females feel the urge to urinate when they participate in making love. It is smart, therefore, for a woman to urinate prior to intercourse.

There are many techniques to stimulate the Mysterious Gate. The simplest way is through direct pressure. You can begin with an increased level of arousal caused by clitoral stimulation. Insert a finger two inches into the vagina and press upward toward the front wall of the vagina. Use one or two fingers, slightly bent; press the anterior wall as you bend and straighten your fingers. This provides pressure and movement against the Mysterious Gate and is basic stimulation. Before doing this, check your fingernails to be sure they are short and smooth. There are also many aspects and functions of the uterus, vagina, and other female sexual anatomy. One of these functions is that they store the negativity caused by abuse a woman has experienced, whether physical or emotional. Arousal and manipulation of the Mysterious Gate can perform the function of releasing this negativity. Such manipulation can be performed by the woman herself or her partner. It needs to be done with the flat portion of the middle fingers or two fingers, just before the

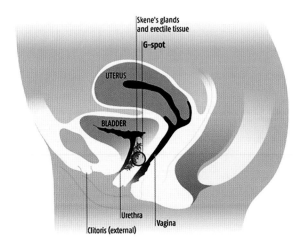

Fig. 5.33. Mysterious Gate is known as the G-spot in the West.

nails. It should not be done with the tips because the nails might cause scratches.

Men often do not have sufficient patience and compassion to bring about a Mysterious Gate orgasm in the woman. A man is often only interested in his own orgasm and, once that is completed, is exhausted and goes to sleep. A large percentage of women have never experienced a Mysterious Gate orgasm and this is quite unfortunate because of the physical and energetic benefits that it can provide. A man needs the patience to bring about a first or second orgasm in the woman. The first orgasm is clitoral and the second is in the Mysterious Gate. The compassion aspect that is required of the man entails allowing the woman to have her orgasm first. A clear understanding of anatomy shows that neither the clitoris nor the Mysterious Gate are exactly built for the penis. Both patience and the proper technique are required to allow the woman to reach orgasm. If both the clitoral and Mysterious Gate orgasm have been attained, it is possible to activate the third gate. In order to open the third gate, the first and

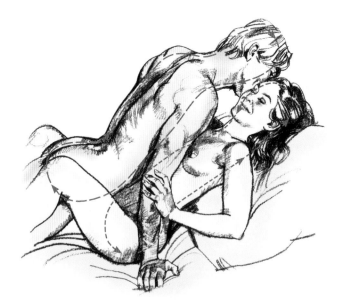

Fig. 5.34. The screwing technique can be done with either the man or the woman in the top position.

second gates must be opened. Otherwise the third gate will remain closed. Once the first two gates are opened, the penis can stimulate the third gate. At this stage the uterus is actually vibrating and contracting. The experience is similar to the reaction a woman has when she is breastfeeding. Achieving the third gate orgasm or what is also called the uterine orgasm reduces the likelihood of getting breast cancer or uterine cancer.

With regard to a woman's orgasm, sacrum training is very important. The sacrum is a triangular bone in the lower back made from fused vertebrae. It is located between the two hipbones of the pelvis. A woman's vagina has to stick to or connect with the sacrum. The same principle applies to a man. If a man's penis sticks to or connects with his sacrum, it is possible for him to rotate his hips correctly in a stirring motion. This motion is very significant in both men and women when it comes to sexual activity. It is a spiraling technique; the sacrum is vital in this activity. This is also often called a screwing technique because of the motion involved (see fig. 5.34). It is not a bumping technique. It can be done with either the man or the woman in the top position.

The screwing technique is actually a sacred dance. Interestingly, the word *sacrum* comes from Latin translation of Greek *hieron osteon* or "sacred bone." It was actually believed that the soul resided there. When the woman is on the top she can feel the penis touching the significant parts of her sexuality. She must have already opened the first and second gates. At that point she can have a uterine orgasm, which is profoundly pleasurable for both the man and the woman.

Simplified Valley Orgasm

1. Make love in any position using a combination of 3 or 9 shallow thrusts (which stimulate the clitoral glans) to 1 deep thrust (which stimulates the cervix), exchanging sexual energy.

2. Upon reaching the point of orgasm, pull penis out until it rests at G-spot. Do gentle Orgasmic Upward Draw with mind power,

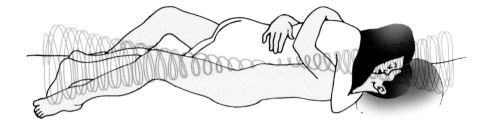

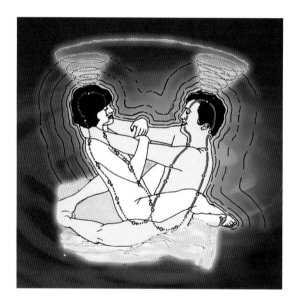

Fig. 5.35. Valley Orgasm and open Microcosmic Orbits in a figure eight

bringing orgasmic energy to the brain, as though it is moving through a valley; exchange sexual energy, with hot male yang energy and cool female yin energy flooding each other's bodies.

3. Embrace and synchronize your breathing. Place yourselves in comfortable positions without undue stress on the limbs. Focus on the rhythm of your partner's energy to unify with them.

4. Stimulate again and follow same procedure, drawing the orgasmic energy to senses (nose, eyes, ears, and tongue), kidneys, spleen, liver, lungs, and heart, healing each other in each section of the body.

5. Open Microcosmic Orbits, directing energy around circuit at all points forming a figure eight connected to partner's mouth and genitals (see fig. 5.35).

6. Exchange orgasms by circulating energy in and around the entwined bodies using meditation fusing on ching (essential energy), shen (spirit), and chi (vital energy), purifying each other.

7. Repeat procedures, continuing after sessions of 81 shallow and 9 deep thrusts (repeat 5 times, that is, 90 thrusts times 5 for 450 thrusts in all).

8. Complete with deep relaxation, absorbing the energy (20 minutes), letting it cool down.

9. Rest, retreat, and collect energy at navel.

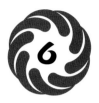

Fusion Alchemy

The understanding of the dynamics of the universe, the planet Earth, and the human body with respect to the five agents of nature (elements or energy phases) and the eight forces of nature is the cornerstone of the Fusion practices. This part of the Tao seeks knowledge and wisdom pertaining to the universe, nature, and humanity. Comprehending Fusion is an interweaving of both the intellect and the energetics (see fig. 6.1).

The fundamental concept to grasp is to realize Fusion collects energy and disperses negativity. The energy is then purified to create chi that can be stored and used to create a healthier and more meaningful life. It proceeds to condense into a pearl of pure energy, which allows the spirit and soul to connect with the universe. The pearl evolves and grows into virtue and consequently creates a more direct relationship with the ultimate forces of the Tao. Channels and bridges are produced to literally move and circulate the chi. Essentially this is a procedure of purification that has the ability to help you to be a better, stronger, and more spiritually mature person.

There are tens of thousands of immortals to call upon. You do not worship these immortals, but rather you ask them to help you. You approach the immortal with respect, honor, and gratitude. There is nothing wrong with asking help from Jesus or any of the other special

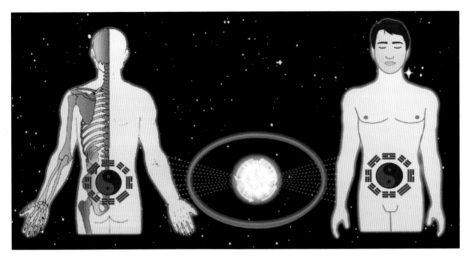

Fig. 6.1. You can fuse with the cosmos and the Tao.

figures from cultures around the world. The point is to request guidance or to be taught in order to move along in your journey toward enlightenment.

FUSION OF THE FIVE ELEMENTS

In our inner universe, our primary organs correspond with the five elements or five phases of energy that are part of the Primordial Force: the kidneys correspond with water, the heart with fire, the liver with wood, the lungs with metal, and the spleen with earth. Due to the alignment of forces in the universe at the time of conception or birth, some people may be born in the condition of being weak or missing some parts of the Primordial Force, causing an imbalance in the body. The Fusion practice combines the energies of the five phases of energy into one harmonious whole. In correspondence to the five elemental forces in nature on Earth, there are dominant forces that affect us from other planets of our solar system. We can balance ourselves by drawing in the appropriate primordial forces from the planets as well: Mars is associated with fire, Mercury with water, and so on.

The bedrock points of Fusion entail all the primary organs of your body, which are interrelated with the internal aspect of yin and yang, responsible for producing energy. The four pakuas are fused in the Fusion of the Five Elements practice. You can consider and comprehend the pakua by starting with the front side of your body and then adding the back, right side, and left side. Being able to focus on one image is of enormous value for the practice of the Tao. If you can picture your pakua you will be able to fuse energy.

It helps to make a copy of the pakua on paper. Make yin blue and yang red (see fig. 6.2). The framework can be black. Then you can place it on the four sides of your body. You can also place it at your feet and at top of the head (six directions). In doing this you are better able to gather and condense chi, which allows you to harmonize better with all the forces of nature. Generally, you should visualize it on the front, both sides, and back, but it is actually all around you.

The energy is transferred to the front pakua, which is viewed as the controlling pakua, then to the back pakua. These two pakuas spiral as

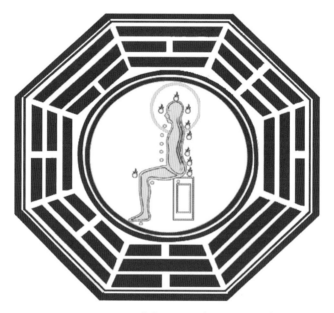

Fig. 6.2. Fusion of the Five Elements—pakua's eight-sided vortex and the Microcosmic Orbit

they draw all the energy into the cauldron, which is located between the navel and the Door of Life, but more toward the back of the body, in front of the kidneys. The pakuas on the right and left sides do the same, as also the top and bottom pakuas. You blend and refine their energy and bring their combined energies into the cauldron. The condensed pakua energy then begins to circulate in the Microcosmic Orbit.

While all this seems complicated, it is not when viewed from the perspective of the connectedness of all things in life. If you use your brain you will be able to grasp this fundamental truth and acquire experience. The experience will give you knowledge and eventually you will acquire wisdom. Wisdom is more than a matter of accumulating facts and information. It is an integral part of the human survival mechanism. The wiser a person becomes, the easier they are able to solve problems and the stronger they become. Their internal army is prepared to balance or neutralize both negativity and illness.

Inner Alchemy of Fusion

Fusion is a matter of gathering and condensing the chi. The center of the brain is always connected to the higher forces (North Star and Big Dipper) through the crown. When you draw the power down, the chi is activated. The alchemy of the Fusion practices will open up the cosmos for you. When they are properly learned and practiced, you will open the gate of spiritual immortality. The connection you open through your crown is like having an antenna on the top of your head to connect to the universe. If you lose your wifi connection, your internet goes down. If you do not have a connection at all, you have no access to the internet. The same can be said of connecting to the universe; practice Fusion and your being will be connected to Ultimate Reality.

As you store and multiply the chi, you will be able to bring even more chi into your being. Your sexual energy has the ability to transform into an energetic force as well as a physical force. This is important because it pertains to an art that seems to have been lost in the West: that of sexual wisdom. The modern world is more sex-driven than ever, but there is a lot of confusion. What we have nowadays is little more than titillation blended with shame. The discussion of sex in the company of others is still an embarrassing notion for many. Many people are even reluctant to discuss sex with those they love. Titillation, secrecy, and wasting sexual power are the unfortunate results of all this confusion.

Once you go beyond the cultural restrictions placed on you, the result will be not only mental health but physical and spiritual health as well (see fig. 6.3). The basics are simple and without immediate sexual connotations. It is about connections to the cosmos and to your body. It is a quest for chi. When approached from a biological, anatomical, and cosmological point of view, it is much easier to think about and share with others. In addition, it is much easier to understand and to relate to in your daily life. It is very pragmatic.

Keep in mind that Taoism is about the two polarities of yin and yang and they are about balance, and you come to a very significant stage of the practice. That stage is balance of the polarities. It is possible to comprehend everything in the universe, from personal things like diet and health to the movement of the planets, in terms of balance.

The process of DNA renewal is critical for health and happiness and a prime mover in the process of creation. Sexual arousal entails both chemistry and vibration. Vibrations are found in the macrocosm as well as the microcosm. The process of making love results in the cells and the DNA cells making love too. The DNA cells actually wrap around each other as though in an embrace. The orgasmic vibration facilitates this embrace and ultimately leads to creation and the birth of new DNA cells. Love is at the foundation of this process. The vibration also extends to the various glands in the body. One of these is the pineal gland, which connects to cosmic energy and helps you extend your axis upward while you are simultaneously connected to Mother Earth.

When the universal forces combine with the energy provided by arousal orgasm, they literally help you overcome death. The result is the creation of your immortal body. The immortal body allows you to leave your physical body consciously when you die. Your spirit will still be energized; it will be immortal because you are transforming material into immaterial and negative into positive. Spiritual energy is the engine that drives the spirit body and brings about Taoist Immortality for a spirit and soul.

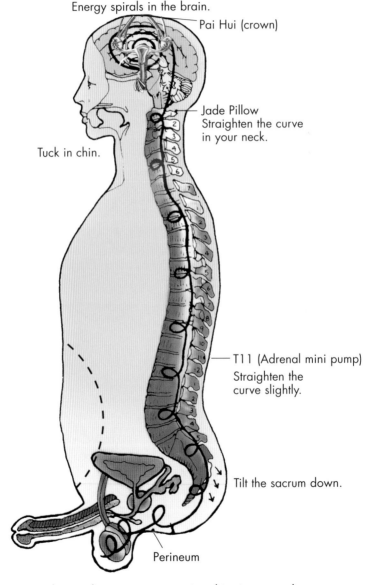

Fig. 6.3. A key to the Taoist practice is cultivating sexual energy.

The central point here is that you increase your energy in the Fusion practices to form a personal energy body. Sexual practices are designed to increase your physical energy so you are healthier and have a life that is happy, healthy, and joyful. Once you get enough energy, you are able to transform it into spiritual energy through Universal Healing Tao sexual practices.

Gathering the Energy in the Hui Yin

As you proceed with your Taoist practice you will have a sensation that the chi is entering your sexual organs. Lift the energy up from Mother Earth and give it permission to enter your body from the area behind the genitals but in front of the anus. As mentioned earlier, this point is known as the Million Dollar point and also known as the Hui Yin or perineum (see fig. 6.4). Visualize the energy collecting there. Be sure to breathe properly as you apply pressure to the Million Dollar point with your fingers. In the beginning for males you will need to do this manually, but with practice, you can do it mentally. Practicing and visualizing will eventually make this virtually automatic. The energy that you summon in this way is inexhaustible sexual energy. The energy will move naturally to your spirit and you will multiply your chi.

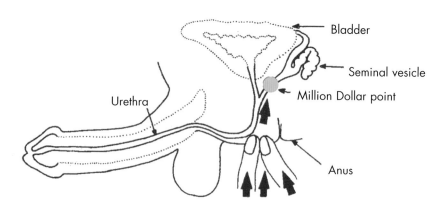

Fig. 6.4. Three-finger press at Hui Yin

After calling upon this energy, you can then proceed to focus on the Tai Chi symbols spinning in your lower abdomen. Visualize all four of them spinning and listen carefully to hear them spin. You will hear the vibration from inside your body. One of the Tai Chi symbols extends down to your sexual organs. Feel the energy spiraling around your glans penis or clitoris. Trust it and you will experience it totally and completely. It is real. Use sexual images if you need help to facilitate the impending orgasm. Then release your entire tension and have your unaroused orgasm. As you have the orgasm, the violet light will enter your being. The violet light is the light of wisdom coming from the Original Force. Sexual energy also comes from the Original Force.

Activate all the bodily glands and wrap them with your orgasm, which connects the physical to the spiritual. The chi will be retained longer in its crystallized state once you master this practice. After you are able to stream energy you will be protected against negative forces in all their manifestations. Once you know how to stream this energy it will slowly become virtually automatic. This is a very powerful energy when it is synthesized and utilized in a manner that entails a balanced approach in accord with the Tao itself. It is the way of nature.

One of the main things to understand is that the Hui Yin is a cross-roads. The front portion connects to your sexual energy. After sexual energy is aroused and multiplied, it must be gathered together. If you do not gather the energy it will run wild throughout your body. The way to stabilize it is to utilize the Hui Yin and the cauldrons (the upper, middle, and lower tan tiens) in your body as collection points. The first step in this practice is to contract the Hui Yin. Then put the tip of your tongue on the roof of the mouth relatively far back. The tongue should be held in place as you do the entire exercise.

Then concentrate on the (lower) tan tien. Feel the energy there. Give your body permission to collect the energy. This is followed by becoming aware of your ovaries or sperm. After you become truly aware of this energy, focus on your Hui Yin. After the energy has completed the gathering stage, it is time to go to the next step of moving on to the coccyx or tailbone. Feel the energy coursing up the spine to the pituitary gland and then to the crown. You utilize your tongue to direct the powerful energy that is contained in your saliva. As it flows back downward it will connect to the navel, tracing your Microcosmic Orbit.

You can sit on a chair with your feet consciously placed on the floor. Focus on the Hui Yin and apply pressure with your fingers. Hold your breath and then exhale. Focus and gather again. Repeat this several times and rock your spine. It should always be loose so you can feel your Fire Dragon. It is a good idea to make a habit of rocking and loosening your spine frequently. This is one process of training your focus and training your Inner Smile. It enables you to access the power. You can literally feel the energy building up internally and you might want to visualize shaping the energy into a ball.

During the practice you must always keep in mind your internal axis connecting not only outward to the universe, but downward to Mother Earth. The earth can be thought of as a large cauldron that is filled with water and produces the steam of life. The soles of your feet are the receptors of the energy that bubbles up from this huge cauldron. It is possible to feel this energy entering your being as you visualize and connect to the earth's forces. You can send a pearl to the earth for the purpose of collecting energy. You need the power on your crown, Hui Yin, and the soles of your feet. That makes your vital connection possible. In this fashion you have sufficient power to move the energy in its flow through the channels of your body.

Hui Yin and Five-Elements Practice

1. Stand up and start by feeling the energy around you as you connect to Mother Earth.
2. Relax your Hui Yin and connect to the earth force.
3. Hold your chin in and become aware of the cosmic force.
4. Feel and visualize the five elements.

5. Connect the cosmic force to Mother Earth down through your crown, the Hui Yin, and the soles of your feet.

6. Connect back up from Mother Earth through your being and into the cosmos.

The mind, spirit, and body operate in conjunction as they extend from Heaven to Earth in a transcendent form of understanding. This is a legitimate inner and subjective feeling, which is essential for the practice. Just as grasping the concepts of yin and yang are vital to Taoist understanding, so too is understanding the connection between yin (Earth) and yang (Heaven). The yin and yang are two parts of one whole, and at the center of yin is yang and at the center of yang is yin. That is clear in the symbol of the Tao.

Yin (Earth) and Yang (Heaven) Practice

1. Fuse your personal chi with the cosmic chi and allow it to multiply.

2. Empty your mind and experience the chi in your bones.

3. Open the point between the thumb and index finger known as the Tiger's Mouth.

4. Activate the energy in your vital organs.

5. Turn the palms of your hands upward and extend them as you draw in the energy.

6. Move the energy into your crown, then down through the cervical vertebrae, clavicle, scapulae, and sternum through your whole being.

7. Be aware of the energy bubbling up from the soles of your feet to the perineum and up your back to the crown.

The practice involves activating your consciousness, awareness, and focus. You must be open and empty when you take in the chi energy. Many people are not connected to their sexual organs in a meaningful way. Being conscious of your energy flow, particularly that emanating from the sexual organs, facilitates your connection to the cosmos. The combination of mental power and personal power allows for a relationship to your creative forces. This involves the power of your consciousness. You are aware, but open. Human beings are aware of the fact that they have energy but often unaware that they leak energy. The leakage is through your sexual organs, negative emotions, and endlessly turning your senses outward with worldly distractions. The senses need to be cleared and balanced and a calm spirit developed. Yin and yang need to be stabilized. The Tao gives you the necessary resources to go beyond the realm of the world of senses. It gives you the means to channel the energy around you.

Chi Transformation with the Pakuas

The eight different sides that make up each pakua are the eight natural forces of the cosmos. First is the force of wind. The second is the thunder, which is followed by the mountain, then water. The heavens make up the fifth force, and the lake the sixth. The seventh force is the earth, and the last one is fire. One function of the pakuas is to draw energy to their spinning centers. This energy becomes the forces of nature, the planets, and the entire cosmos. You need to remember to spin these forces in order to properly align and expel negativity while bringing in the positive forces of Mother Earth and nature itself (see fig. 6.5).

When the pakuas spin they expand outward first to nature and then to the universe. Then they draw the forces inward when you place your mind into the center of your body or tan tien. You experience your being and spin. Your body spins at first as you look downward. As you begin to spin faster and faster, you expand more and more. You can start with the Inner Smile in the front pakua and think about your internal organs. Look inward and see the connection with all your organs. Move from one organ to another as you heal and spin. You can use your sexual energy to restore and revitalize each vital organ: your kidneys, heart, lungs, liver, and spleen.

As you spiral in your front and back pakuas, then with the right

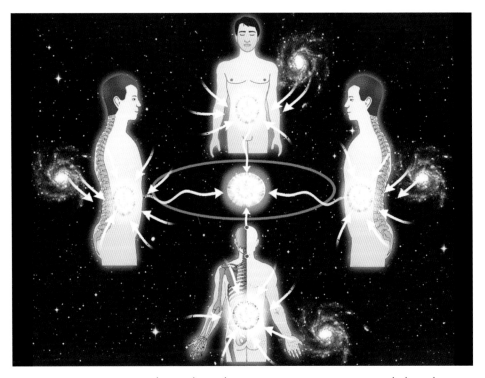

Fig. 6.5. Activate and spin the pakuas on your torso. Be sure to link to the center because this is the Source.

and left pakuas, let go of sadness, cruelty, anger, fear, and worry. Move on to your crown and open it as violet light comes to your brain. The crown is connected to the front pakua. The brain and all the organs use the power of aroused orgasmic energy. Draw energy from the sexual arousal as you draw it through your crown. You are utilizing both inner and outer forces to energize yourself. Condense the energy at the navel. Chi fills your saliva and has power in the same way water has power. Use the saliva and circulate it in the Microcosmic Orbit. Touch your navel with your fingertips and swallow. You may belch as the chi replaces negative forces. Do not be shy if this takes place, because it is healthy. The four pakuas form the chi that you hold on to with the mind, spirit, soul, and heart.

You spin the Tai Chi the same speed as the earth spins. Make sure to be totally aware of everything. Feel everything and know your body, spirit, and soul. Take in the forces from the different sides of your body and move them to the center of your body. Hold the chi there. Keep in mind that chi comes and chi goes, and consequently you must focus in order to hold it. Know the significant regions of your body and the locations of the pakuas.

Many of the practices are repeated at various points. The basic concept as you proceed is to create something from nothing. Your mind, eyes, and heart need to be quite focused. Once you have achieved this, you can then begin to gather the chi. When your spirit and soul come together, you will then have the power. At that point you will have wisdom and be well on the path toward both physical and philosophical enlightenment. You will have accomplished this yourself because the source of enlightenment is found in all sentient beings.

At this stage you can create a chi ball. A chi ball is a simple yet useful tool for directing and expanding your healing energy and protective energy throughout your entire body. Your own personal energy constitutes the chi ball; once you master this very important practice you are in control of the energy that constitutes this powerful force. It assists in facilitating both centering and grounding your being. In addition, it provides strong forces against negativity and illness. You are giving yourself a shield to maintain and refresh your chi.

You start by focusing on the area around your navel and bringing your breath into your abdomen. This is abdominal breathing. Make sure that you are connected to Mother Earth and maintain your strong belief in the practice. Remain focused and become one with the eternal Tao. You can utilize any of the symbols that have been discussed to help you stay centered, such as the yin and yang symbol, colors, the Eight Immortals, or something of your own choosing. Make sure to breathe and relax as you do this. You should have a pleasant sensation akin to contentment at this stage.

Simplified Fusion of the Five Elements

 Formula 1: Forming Four (or Six) Pakuas and Pearl

1. In sitting position, eyes closed, do Inner Smile.
2. Turn awareness and senses inward toward the navel, feeling warmth and forming energy ball.
3. Look inward 1.5 inches inside navel. With mind power, draw the first line of the pakua.
4. Continue doing all eight lines of the outer layer of pakua, then do the second layer one line at a time, then the third, inner layer.
5. Draw eight spokes from outer to inner layer, then Tai Chi symbol in middle (see fig. 6.6). Spiral the pakua, which blends and transforms energy, feeling the pakua glowing with white light.
6. Follow same procedure to form back pakua at Door of Life, then

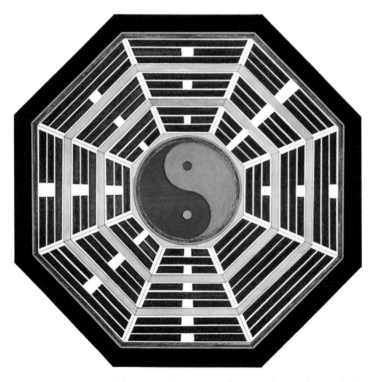

Fig. 6.6. Fusion of the Five Elements pakua and Tai Chi symbol

spiral both pakuas, drawing energy into the cauldron, condensing light while rocking the spine.

7. Follow same procedure for right and left side pakuas, below armpit and level with navel. You can also form pakuas at top (crown) and bottom (below feet at soles). Spiral energy into cauldron while rocking the spine.

8. In relaxed manner continue spiraling into cauldron, forming the pearl, drawing all essence of your organs, glands, senses, and mind into pure energy. Feel pearl become stronger and brighter, grounding, centering, and balancing you, while rocking the spine.

9. Move pearl in Microcosmic Orbit, concentrating at each point, becoming aware of the North Star and Big Dipper (violet/red light), cosmic force (golden light), and earth force (blue light), drawing in from crown, mid-eyebrow, and perineum.

❷ Formula 2: Balancing Inner Climate

1. Form front pakua and kidneys collection point at perineum by doing kidneys' sound: choo-oo-oo-oo (as when blowing out a candle), packing kidneys, drawing any cold energy of the body into a blue ball at perineum.

2. Relax. Follow same procedure with heart collection point, drawing energy into a red ball at sternum with heart's sound: haw-w-w-w-w-w.

3. Spiral into front pakua the blue and red balls, drawing in cold blue energy and hot red energy blending into one energy.

4. Follow same procedure, drawing the energies of your liver and lungs into a green ball (warm and moist energy) below liver and white ball (dry and cool energy) on left side opposite liver, and draw them into front pakua.

5. Follow same procedure for back pakua, then spiral and draw energy, condensing it into cauldron; then add right and left pakuas (and top and bottom if you wish), refining pearl in cauldron while rocking the spine. Relax.

6. Feel at peace and an inner harmony creating a perfect internal climate: not too hot, cold, moist, or dry. Send pearl in orbit.

⊘ Formula 3: Connecting Senses and Organ

1. Massage ears and kidneys, spiraling any sounds to kidneys. Draw sense of hearing to kidney collection point at perineum (blue ball) then move tongue, connecting to heart's energy (sense of speech), to heart's collection point at sternum (red ball), then spiral both kidney and heart energy into front pakua and feel hot and cold energies blending sounds, rocking the spine.

2. Do same procedure for eyes and liver and nose and lungs. Feel moist, warm (sense of sight) and dry, cool (sense of smell) energies blending in front pakua; feel mild energy of mouth and spleen (sense of taste) in yellow ball at navel.

3. Form back, right, and left pakuas (and top and bottom if you wish), and spiral into cauldron; feel a sense of control with "I am calm, clear, at peace, centered in physical and emotional balance."

⊘ Formula 4: Transforming Negative Emotions

1. Turn attention toward ears and be aware of any fear sensations (chilling, cloudy blue, awkward shapes) listening to kidneys. Spiral and breathe any fear out of the kidneys into a blue ball at kidney collection point at the perineum (see fig. 6.7 on page 256).

2. Move tongue and be aware of any cruelty sensations (hot, muddy red, unsteady, acidic) in heart. Spiral and breathe any cruelty out into a red ball at heart collection point at sternum.

3. Spiral, blend, and transform negative energy of the kidney and heart collection points (blue and red balls) in front pakua.

4. Move eyes and perceive anger sensations (steamy, murky green, sharp spear) in liver. Spiral and breathe any anger out into a green ball at liver collection point below the liver.

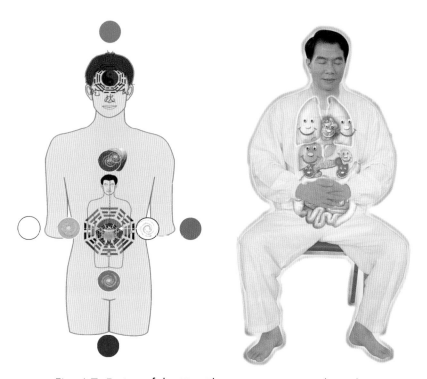

Fig. 6.7. Fusion of the Five Elements—setting up the pakuas,
pearl, and negative emotions

5. Inhale and exhale and be aware of sadness sensations (brisk, gray, musty, salty) in lungs. Spiral and breathe any sadness out into a white ball at lung collection point opposite liver.

6. Spiral, blend, and transform negative energy of liver and lung's green and white balls into front pakua, while rocking the spine.

7. Move lips and be aware of any worry sensations (sticky yellow, uncertain, souring) in spleen. Spiral and breathe any worry out into a yellow ball at spleen collection point at navel.

8. Spiral, blend, and transform (act of forgiveness) all remaining negative energy into front pakua. Focus inwardly to sounds, sights, smells, and tastes, and feel virtue energies and qualities of prosperity, willpower, vitality, decisiveness, and stability grow.

9. Form back, right, and left pakuas (and top and bottom if you wish)

and draw energies into cauldron, spiraling and breathing in and out, forming pearl.

10. Move pearl to perineum and circulate in Microcosmic Orbit.

COSMIC FUSION

Chanting the sounds of the Tao is the love song of your DNA. As you do any of the chanting, it is important to create some vibration because the cosmos vibrates. You can think of this almost like a tuning fork. We communicate not just with other people through our vibrations but with the cosmos itself. You can chant the directions as follows: *li - kan - chen - tui - sun - chien - kun - ken*. The eight sounds sing about the crossing of the chromosomes that wrap around each other over and over. They are making love. Another way to do it is to use the special sounds advocated by ancient Taoist practitioners:

Wood: Sh-h-h-h-h-h, pronounced like sh in the word "hush"
Fire: Haw-w-w-w-w-w, like haw in the word "hawk"
Earth: Who-oo-oo-oo-oo, just like the word "who"
Metal: Sss-s-s-s-s-s, very quietly, pronounced "seeee-ah"
Water: Choo-oo-oo-oo-oo, rounding the lips and silently making the sound you make when blowing out a candle

There are other sounds, too; all should be regarded as chants and done in a serious way. Make the connections to the inner you and your organs. Every aspect of the universe has its own special characteristics and is connected to all the other cosmic entities. One of those entities is you. Chanting connects you to the universe. It is a healing process. Trust that you can make the inner and outer connections and it will happen. Trusting is not only seeing but involves all the senses of your body. The results of this line of thinking can even be seen in the binary mathematics used with computers. The yin and yang symbol with the broken lines and the solid lines is essentially a binary formation. You can see that Taoist chanting has millions of formations.

Chanting reunites the elements with your internal being. Then you can reunite all the natural forces with your true self. This unification or reunion is of yourself, nature, and the universe. Symbols have power and words have power. When you put the symbol and the word together, you have the power. Visualize the yin and yang symbol and, as you chant each line of the different trigrams, visualize the power of the word, power of the symbol, and power of the chant connecting to the ultimate power of the universe.

Chanting starts with the lower tan tien and the vocal cords. The entire connection between the tan tien and the crown of your head is used in chanting. You commence with the lower tan tien, activate with the sound in the vocal cords (see fig. 6.8), and ultimately use the antenna on your crown to move out into the cosmos and make a universal connection.

As you chant you are calling all the forces of the universe. You can think of four of the trigrams as below and have a good idea of all eight directions.

Yin, yin, yin is the earth and is receptive, which is verbalized "by the power of the earth."

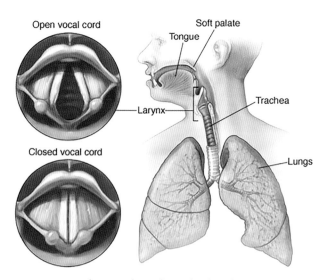

Fig. 6.8. The vocal cords and related organs

Yang, yin, yin is the mountain and is stillness, which is verbalized "by the power of the mountain."

Yin, yang, yin is the water and is immeasurable, which is verbalized "by the power of water."

Yang, yang, yin is the wind and is gentle, which is verbalized "by the power of wind."

Visualize the different trigrams as you chant them to make them more powerful (see fig. 6.9). Extend the sound like this: "kaaaaaahn."

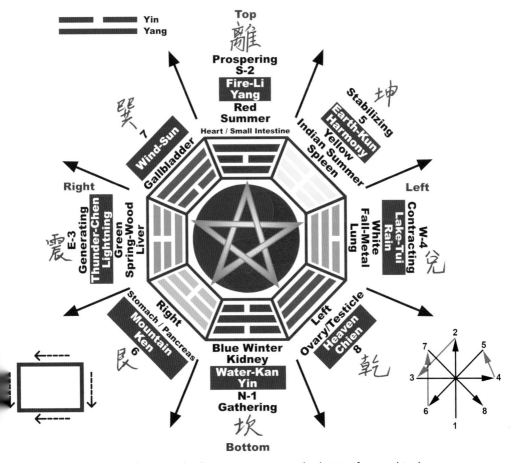

Fig. 6.9. Start chanting the lowest trigram marked N-1 (for north), then go to the top, S-2, and continue on, following the sequence of the numbers. Note that a broken line is yin and a solid line is yang.

Start the sound from the associated part of your body. Start with a deeper tone, then extend it for about five seconds while going to a slightly higher tone. Moving around the yin and yang directions of your body will connect you to all the different elements of nature. As you make the connections you will ultimately be connected to the highest power; that is, the Tao, God, or whatever name you choose to associate with this power.

Chanting the Trigrams

Chanting the names of the different trigrams related to the directions begins with chanting the name of the trigram, followed by chanting the lines of the trigram. Start in the lower part of your body, the lower tan tien or *yin, yang, yin.* Do each step in order:

Kan: *yin, yang, yin*
Li: *yang, yin, yang*
Chen: *yin, yin, yang*
Tui: *yin, yang, yang*
Kun: *yin, yin, yin*
Ken: *yang, yin, yin*
Sun: *yang, yang, yin*
Chien: *yang, yang, yang*

Continue until you can feel the spinning of the Tai Chi in the area of your abdomen. This practice has been used for thousands of years. It has been practiced by millions of people and has worked for those who do the practice right and trust in the practice. There is no substitute for actually hearing the sounds of the chanting, so it is best to contact a reputable instructor or to find a source on the internet (www.universal -tao.com) that you are sure is legitimate. If you have ever heard actual monks chanting, you have some concept of how the chant might sound, but it is best to seek out an expert.

Visualization is also very important in order to do this practice properly. You need to open all the senses so that there is true unification. As the sounds are burned into your being you can actually feel the warmth and smell the burning process. Use your eyes and see the different forces. You can see the water, thunder, wind, fire, earth, heaven, lake, and mountain forces. You can see the Eight Immortals and colors.

Think in terms of gathering the forces of nature and moving on to gather the forces of the universe. Keep in mind that you are utilizing these powerful dynamic forces. They are the foundation of the Fusion practice. Internally you can activate the Primordial Force and align yourself with nature. Once you get this practice down well, you will find it quite easy to activate with a simple act of your will.

Opening the Channels

The Cosmic Fusion practice is a method of strengthening your connection to the cosmos. The different channels in your body are essential in order to attain this connection. The channels are the Thrusting Channels, Belt Channels, and the Regulator and Bridge Channels. The channels are responsible for protecting the body and regulating its energy. Fusion of the Five Elements connects to the primordial forces in the pakuas. Then the negative energy is cleansed from your organs and a pearl is formed, which circulates the energy in the Microcosmic Orbit. Cosmic Fusion opens your Thrusting and Belt Channels (see fig. 6.10 on page 262). This fuses your positive energy and charges you with additional chi.

Your Thrusting Channels are something you should be very aware of for several reasons. They are essentially the major energy routes in your body. Running vertically, they connect the cosmos with the earth's energy, establishing a vital connection for your life. These routes detoxify and energize your vital organs.

The Belt Channels wrap around the other channels and hold them together like a cylinder. They start in the area of the navel and spiral

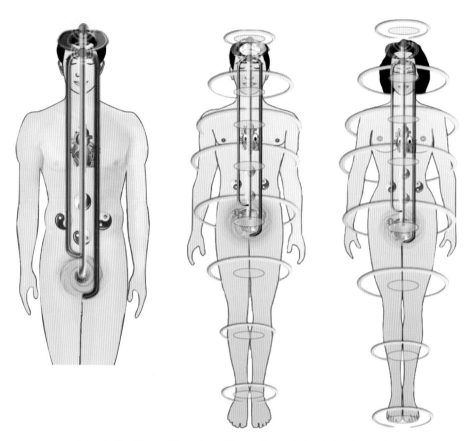

Fig. 6.10. Three Thrusting Channels and the Belt Channels

counterclockwise in an upward direction. They transfer the energy to the various other channels, which set up protection for the body's centers. This combats external negative energy.

Cosmic Fusion practice opens the Thrusting Channels and improves awareness. As your understanding and vision broadens, you can see that your being has all the necessary tools to collect, store, and maintain the energy that you need for a positive existence. Opening the various channels involves building up energy. The only place to acquire that energy is from the sexual organs, because only sexual energy can be stored and utilized.

The place to start is with the Hui Yin, which connects to the crown.

The perineum, or Gate of Life and Death, is the primary foundation for sexual energy. The energy from Mother Earth is collected in this location and then goes on to connect to the other channels in the body. The Central Thrusting Channel runs upward from the Hui Yin to the crown and is of critical importance (see fig. 6.11). It has the function of regulating the flow of energy and keeping it in balance. It regulates the flow of your blood and fights infections. Opening this channel promotes the free flow of energy in your body. It prepares your body to gain and accept a higher form of energy with the power of immortality. As the energy flows into your body, it spreads outward, cleansing and rejuvenating all the organs in your body. As it spreads it creates energy that can be stored for use by your energetic self.

The Middle Channel has a yin and a yang element. Meridians of the organs control the flow of energy. The yang part is responsible

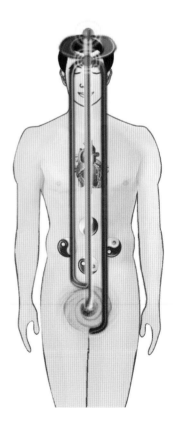

Fig. 6.11. The Middle or Central Thrusting Channel running from the Hui Yin to the crown is of critical importance.

for connecting the yang meridians and controlling that portion of the energy flow. Yin channels regulate the blood while yang channels regulate resistance to infection. In this way the yin is an offensive mechanism while yang is a defensive mechanism. You can think of it as an alchemical vision of the way the body works. Regardless of how you understand it, this theory has met the test of time for thousands of years.

To open the channels, first concentrate on your energy flow. You need to feel this flow in the channels. You can use your hands and your mind to help with awareness. Visualize or touch the various points on your body where the energy is flowing: through your face, the front of the body, and the interior part of the legs, then moving on to your hips and spine, then your shoulders and armpits, including your arms and neck. Repetition is important so that you can go on to the capability of almost automatic activation.

You exhale and release all negativity and then breathe in. Open your crown, using your hand if necessary to apply pressure to the top of your head. If you do not know the precise point, that is not an issue. Simply do the best you can and your body will inform you of the right places. You can utilize this to open your inner Thrusting Channels as well as the protective Belt Channels. Energy circles expand the reach of the Primordial Force.

Start the process of activation by breathing and expanding your energy in your midsection. Proceed to notice the spinning of the energy. This is essentially a mirror of what takes place in the universe. As it is on the inside, so it is on the outside. Spiral the energy upward to the throat and middle eyebrow, then spiral it back down to the sexual organs, perineum, knees, and soles of the feet. As you improve and increase this process, your health and healing powers are increased. You are able to develop spiritually to a greater degree. Spiritual energy is the primary component relative to immortality in the Taoist philosophy.

At this stage, you must open the more protective channels. This takes place in your spine and head as well as throughout your body.

At this juncture you are at a place where refining and protecting your energy body is taking place. It is a critical phase. You are at a place where almost total rejuvenation and refreshing of energy channels in your body is possible because you can open your Bridge and Regulator Channels. You have additional esoteric protection and can purge yourself of bodies that negatively impact your spine and brain. All of this means that you can circulate vital energy much more effectively. This is the key to physical and spiritual health and is one of the most significant teachings of the ancient Taoist masters.

The Cosmic Fusion practice teaches additional methods of circulating the pure energy of the five organs once they are freed of negative emotions. When the five organs are cleansed, the positive emotions of kindness, gentleness, respect, fairness, justice, and love are combined into pearls of compassion energy that emerge as a natural expression of internal balance. We use the master pakua "energy transforming factory" to produce these positive chi pearls, which are then used to open the inner Thrusting Channels and the outer protective Belt Channels. We also work with energy circles to broaden the range of Primordial Force access and protection. This is part of the process of forming our energy body vehicle for gathering more Primordial Force for health, healing, and spiritual development.

Simplified Cosmic Fusion

Formula 1: Creation Channel (Growing Virtues)

1. Be aware of kidneys and do kidneys' sound (choo-oo-oo-oo), drawing cold energy to kidney collection point, listening to gentleness growing to form a big blue ball at perineum (see fig. 6.12 on page 266).
2. Look to liver with liver's sound (sh-h-h-h-h-h), as gentleness gives birth to kindness and moist energy in liver collection point, forming a big green ball on the right side; feel it expand.

3. Feel tongue connect with heart and do heart's sound (haw-w-w-w-w-w). Gentleness and kindness give birth to joy, growing hot energy in heart collection point, forming a big red ball in upper body.

4. Feel mouth connect with spleen, doing spleen's sound (who-oo-oo-oo). Gentleness, kindness, and joy give birth to fairness, growing mild energy in spleen collection point into big yellow ball, expanding it in the center of body.

5. Feel nose connect with lungs and do lungs' sound (sss-s-s-s-s-s). Gentleness, kindness, joy, and fairness give birth to courage in lung collection point, a big white ball on left side.

6. Creation Cycle: Complete cycle from kidney to lung collection points, combining virtue pearls and growing virtues to heal the body. Repeat the cycle and blend virtues each time by growing the pearls in all collection points (9 times).

7. Compassion Energy: Blend all virtue energies into golden compassion pearl. Move pearl in creation cycle (kidneys–liver–heart–spleen–lungs)

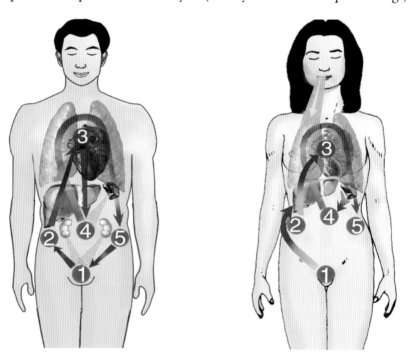

Fig. 6.12. Cosmic Fusion—Creation Channel

3–6 times. Stop at heart and feel virtues flow, glow, and expand in heart. Feel heart open and blend virtues into compassion energy. Feel sexual arousal flow into heart, activating compassion, then move pearl to cauldron and form bigger compassion pearl, then move pearl in the Microcosmic Orbit, loving and healing the organs.

🜨 Formula 2: Thrusting Channels

In this practice, you need to clearly visualize the movement of the pearl through the three Thrusting Channels (see fig. 6.13 on page 268):

Left Thrusting (Red) Channel: Move pearl to left anus, left genital, left kidney, spleen, left lung, left thyroid, left brain.
Middle Thrusting (White) Channel: Move pearl to anus, cervix or prostate, pancreas, heart, throat, pineal gland, and crown.
Right Thrusting (Blue) Channel: Move pearl to right anus, right genital, right kidney, liver, right lung, and right brain.

1. Inhale pearl with left nostril up left (red) channel to diaphragm. Exhale down left channel to perineum.
2. Inhale up middle (white) channel to crown. Exhale down middle channel to perineum.
3. Inhale pearl with right nostril up right (blue) channel to crown. Exhale down right channel to perineum.
4. Continue in middle, left, middle, right, middle, and left (9 times).

🜨 Leg Routes

1. **Men:** Bring pearl from perineum up and out of crown (6 inches), absorbing heavenly energy, shooting pearl down channels from legs to toes into the earth, drawing earth energy up through sole up to crown (9 times).
   Women: Reverse, from crown to soles out into the crown, gathering the heavenly force.

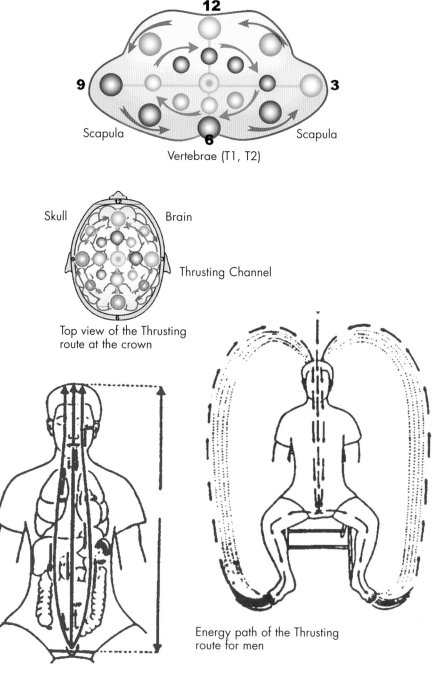

Lung Thrusting Channel

12

9

3

Scapula

6

Scapula

Vertebrae (T1, T2)

Skull

Brain

Thrusting Channel

Top view of the Thrusting route at the crown

Energy path of the Thrusting route for men

Fig. 6.13. Cosmic Fusion—Thrusting Channels

☢ *Formula 3: Belt Channels*

1. Circulate pearl counterclockwise from left side to Door of Life, to right side, then back to navel, 9 times, then crisscross.

2. Move pearl to the left side of each of the following positions: solar plexus, heart, throat, mid-eye, crown, halo (6 inches) above head; at each level circulate pearl counterclockwise 9 times, then crisscross.

3. At halo, move pearl clockwise from front to right, back, left, and front (9 times), then crisscross.

4. Move pearl to the right side of each of the following positions: crown, mid-eye, throat, heart, solar plexus, navel, sexual center, perineum, knees, soles, beneath the earth (6 inches); at each level circulate pearl clockwise 9 times, then crisscross.

5. Reverse the circle beneath the earth, moving the pearl counterclockwise 9 times and then crisscross; repeat at soles, knee, perineum, sexual center, navel, and return to cauldron.

6. Breathe, shoot pearl out (6 inches) above crown; collect heavenly energy, spiral pearl (clockwise) down each Belt Channel into the earth (12 inches), then reverse spiraling (counterclockwise), gathering earth energy up each channel to crown, back to navel, up and down, using the body as a pipe from Earth to Heaven (9 times).

FUSION OF EIGHT PSYCHIC CHANNELS

Fusion of the Eight Psychic Channels teaches the final techniques and meditations needed to prepare you for the higher practices of the Immortal Tao. Fusion of the Eight Psychic Channels includes: opening and cleaning the Great Bridge and the Great Regulator Channel; learning to protect your spine and energy field, clear your senses, drill your head with energy, and seal your aura; learning to form an energy body and transfer the Microcosmic Orbit, the Thrusting Channels, and the Belt Channels to it.

The channels are both receivers and distributors of the universal force. The Regulator Channels simply prevent your energy from becoming too hot or cold. They regulate the energy as it moves through your body. The Bridge Channels make connections to other channels, making it possible for the energy to stream in any direction and provide chi to all parts of your body. Each channel has its own distinct functions. The Great Bridge Channel facilitates the flow of chi among the various meridians while the Great Regulator Channel connects and balances the flow as it spreads to the different meridians. In this manner all the meridians act together and enable the energy to flow from one meridian to another.

The Great Bridge and Regular Channels have both a yin and a yang component. The yin channels establish connection among the yin organs and the yang does this for the yang organs. The yin channels are found on the inside of the arms and legs as well as the front of the body (see fig. 6.14). The yang channels are located on the outside of the arms and legs as well as the back of the body (see fig. 6.15 on page 272). Yin is associated with defending against internal issues and yang defends the body against external attacks. Opening the Bridge and Regulator Channels prevents blockages of energy, thus healing and receiving quality energy. Knowing how to utilize these channels can protect the spine and assist with energetic aspects of your being. Utilizing these channels properly can help regulate, coordinate, and balance chi in your meridians.

A number of points in the Universal Healing Tao Fusion practice are significant because they allow for the flow of energy throughout your body to promote health and longevity. The Gall Bladder meridian is located behind the center on the top area of your cranium and to the left and right sides. It moves up on the head, down the back, and through the facial region near the eyebrow. As you do the practice you need to be aware of various parts of your cranium as you circulate the energy. Concentrate, visualize, and trust.

The remaining meridians are the Stomach meridian, Liver meridian, Spleen meridian, Heart meridian, Pericardium meridian, Triple Warmer meridian, Kidney meridian, Bladder meridian, Small Intestine meridian, Lung meridian, and Large Intestine meridian. It is important to gain

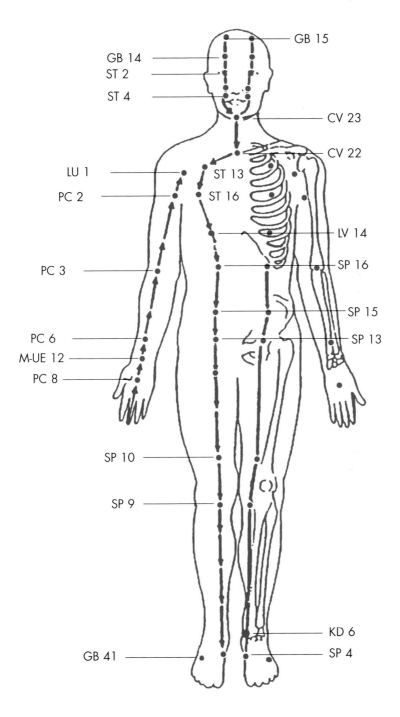

Fig. 6.14. The yin side of the body

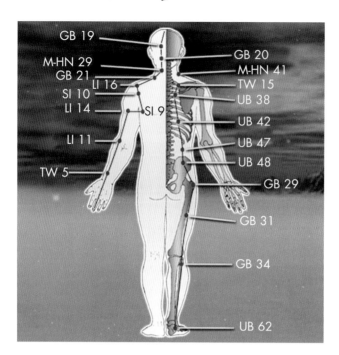

Fig. 6.15.
The yang side
of the body

significant familiarity with the human anatomy. This includes the internal organs and their relationships to the various points of your body. Those points include your back as well as major joints like your knees and elbows. Studying anatomy along with your practices of the Tao is highly recommended.

An essential function of Cosmic Fusion is to assist in the growth of the pearl to open up the channels, which aids in the increase of good virtue. Positive chi purifies your essence and inspires improved control of the forces within you. You are able to create a life force that is purer and the result of better self-control. The Fusion of the Five Elements is also an integral part of this process. You can sit or stand as you smile down while fusing the five elements. After this you need to reactivate the pakuas with special attention to your face as you connect to the universal pakua. You spiral as you draw the energy into your organs and then the cauldron located in your lower tan tien, making sure your emotions are balanced so that your compassion will be able to expand.

You condense your energy and move the pearl down to the

perineum, connecting to Mother Earth and taking in these forces as you connect upward to the universe. You will feel the energy and you will also note the transcendent nature of the experience. You use your perineum to cleanse the left (red), middle (white), and right (blue) sections of your Thrusting Channels. The pearl is moved up and down through all three Thrusting Channels to the crown. As you breathe, you inhale and pull in the positive energy and exhale all the negative forces. All three Thrusting Channels are purged of toxins and negativity.

Then when you focus on your center you will feel the chi gathering there. You will notice the increase in the positive forces of the universe brought to you from opening the channels. The feeling is real. The procedure is essentially the same for each channel. Repetition makes the practice easier and eventually it will become automatic and easy to activate. The universe contains negative forces and those forces can manifest themselves as bad spirits or negative energy. This interpretation is applied and initiated by you. Essentially, if you approach the world with a positive perspective, the negative forces—in whatever form you visualize and interpret them—are neutralized. That is why practices like the Inner Smile and clearing of the Thrusting and Belt Channels are so important. They disperse negative energy or spirits.

The Universal Healing Tao practice is based on the principle that the mind, body, and spirit work in conjunction; they are connected and form one totality. This totality is the Eternal Tao. The sexual organs are part of this unity and the source of your life force. The Taoist sexual practices generate hormonal and nervous energy. The additional energy that has the potential to be generated can be channeled throughout the body. It can rejuvenate and increase your energetic and physical powers. The embrace of a man and woman allows for yin and yang energy to be shared, creating a finer balance and an atmosphere of love, joy, and happiness.

However, the sexual organs cannot store energy in an efficient manner. Your brain has the ability to draw in the higher forces and store the additional energy. With time and practice the brain has the ability to convert sexual energy into usable protein. Among the benefits is an improved connection between the nerve cells, especially those in the central nervous system.

Fusion of the Eight Psychic Channels completes the cleansing of the energy channels in the body. The chi pearls are used to open and connect the Bridge and Regulator Channels, and then open more protective channels for the spine, head, and body. These are all used to further refine and protect the energy body. In this level you build extra psychic protection and learn techniques to drive out negative energy entities that attach to the spine and other areas. There are specialized practices to protect the spine and to clear the brain.

The opening of the Microcosmic Orbit, the Thrusting Channels, the Belt Channels, and the Great Regulator and Bridge Channels makes the body extremely permeable to the circulation of vital energy. The unhindered circulation of energy is the foundation of perfect physical and emotional health. The Fusion practice is one of the greatest achievements of the ancient Taoist masters, as it gives the individual a way of freeing the body of negative emotions and, at the same time, allows the pure virtues to shine forth.

 ## Simplified Fusion of the Eight Psychic Channels

Refer to figure 6.14 on page 271 and figure 6.15 on page 272 for point locations.

🌀 *Formula 1: Great Regulator and Bridge Channels*

1. Draw pearl to perineum and split into two pearls, then inhale them up left (red) and right (blue) Thrusting Channels.
2. Draw pearls up to GB 16 (middle side crown points).
3. Exhale shooting pearls out to GB 17 (back crown points, located 3 cun behind GB 15), to GB 16 (on both sides 1.5 cun behind GB 15), to GB 15 (front crown points), then down to GB 14 (just above eyebrows).

4. Down to ST 2 (below eyes) and ST4 (above lips).

5. To CV 23 (under chin) to CV 22 (throat).

6. To ST 13 (below collarbone) and ST 16 (at ribs); LV 14 (at lower ribs), then to SP 16 (abdomen), SP 15, and SP 13.

7. To SP 10 and SP 9 (above and below inside of knees).

8. To KD 6 (inside heel) and SP 4 (inside lower feet).

9. To KD 1 (underneath feet) and GB 41(outside of feet).

10. To UB 62 (under outside of ankles), GB 34 (outside below knees), GB 31 (outside of thighs), GB 29 (inside of hip points), and UB 48 (inside of hip bones).

11. Up back to UB 47 (both sides), UB 42 (T 11), UB 38 (wing points) to TW 15 (upper scapula) and back to UB 42.

12. Up to SI 10 (back of shoulder) and SI 9 (back of shoulder), down outside of arms to LI 14 and LI 11.

13. To back of wrist TW 5 (Triple Warmer), to PC 8 (palms), to MU-E 12 (inside of wrist), to PC 6 (inner arm), to PC 3 (inside elbows), to PC 2 and LU 1 (in- and outside of armpits).

14. To LU I 16 (shoulder points), then up to GB 21, M-HN 41, and M-HN 29 (neck points), to Jade Pillow, GB 20, and GB 19.

15. Connect with crown points and do cycle with breath, feeling energy movement opening up all meridians (9 times).

☯ Formula 2: Spinal Cutting

1. Inhale, exhale, and project the pearl out from the throat (see fig. 6.16A on page 276). Orbit it around the outside of your head to the back and continue the orbit so that the pearl penetrates or "cuts" through your body to C7. Bring the pearl through C7 and project it out through the front of your body.

2. Continue orbiting the pearl in progressively larger loops to cut through each of your cervical, thoracic, and lumbar vertebrae, then down through your sacrum and coccyx (24 times).

3. Finish by bringing pearl back to throat center.

❂ Formula 3: Spinal Microcosmic Orbit

1. Bring pearl down into the sacrum and run it up the back side of and around the spinal cord, twisting up into the brain (see fig. 6.16B).
2. Wrap pearl around frontal lobe inside skull.
3. Return it down inside and in front of the spine, wrapping it around the length of the whole spine. Bring pearl into spinal cord, change directions, direct it down back of spinal cord to sacrum.
4. Wrap pearl around coccyx, bringing energy up front of spine to frontal lobe, then wrap pearl around skull and down backside of spine to the mid-brain (3 times).

❂ Formula 4: Aura Cutting

1. Move pearl to mid-eye using eyes to cut through sides of neck (clockwise or counterclockwise) (see fig. 6.16C).

A. Spinal Cutting   B. Spinal Microcosmic Orbit   C. Aura Cutting

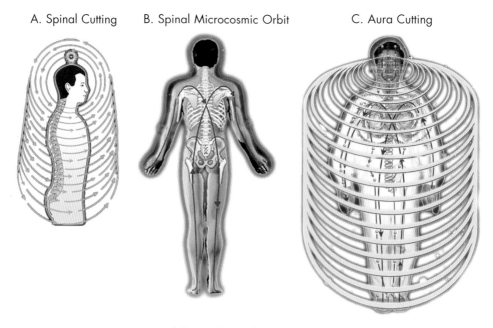

Fig. 6.16. Fusion of the Eight Psychic Channels—Spinal Cutting, Spinal Microcosmic Orbit, and Aura Cutting

2. Cut aura a little lower each time until whole body has been cut and return to mid-eye (20 times).

🌀 Formula 5: Crown Drilling into Head, Opening Crown

1. Move pearl to mid-eye and drill by spiraling pearl into head vertically to base of skull from point to point around the crown (see fig. 6.17a on page 278).
2. Drill pearl all over head to opposite points (3 times).

🌀 Formula 6: Cutting the Senses

1. Move pearl to mid-eye (½ inch inside skull) then move pearl in three figure eights around sense openings (see fig. 6.17b on page 278).
2. From mid-eye around upper right eye, under lower right ear, around upper right ear, under lower right eye, over upper left eye, under lower left ear, around upper left ear, under lower left eye, down right side of nose, under nose, around left side of mouth, under mouth, around right side of mouth, up left side of nose to mid-eye (3 times).

🌀 Formula 7: Heart Center Cutting, Protecting Aura

1. Move pearl to heart collection point at the sternum.
2. Split pearl into two pearls and spiral them cutting through heart center in outward and downward arcs like butterfly wings (right pearl clockwise and left pearl counterclockwise) (see fig. 6.17c on page 278).
3. Spirals grow larger each time, forming body's aura shield (20 times).

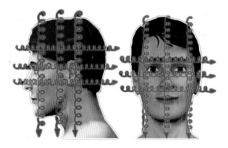

A. Crown Drilling

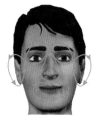

B. Cutting the Senses

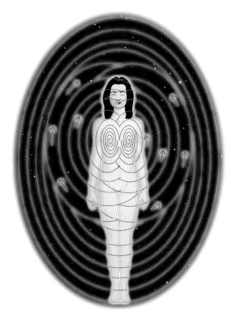

C. Heart Center Cutting

Fig. 6.17. Fusion of the Eight Psychic Channels—
Crown Drilling, Cutting the Senses, and Heart Center Cutting

🌀 Formula 8: Sealing the Aura

1. Re-form pearl at cauldron with six pakuas and move pearl down inside of right leg to right big toe (see fig. 6.18).

2. Jump pearl to left big toe and spread it, outlining body sides, tracing left toes, outside of left leg, up left side to left armpit, down inside left arm, then fingers up outside left arm over left shoulder and crown.

3. Trace down right shoulder, then outside of right arm and fingers, up inside of right arm, then down right side and outside of right leg to toes. Trace toes, then up inside of right leg around genitals, down inner left leg to left big toe.

4. Jump pearl to right big toe and reverse tracing right to left.

5. Then jump pearl from right big toe to left big toe and flatten pearl. Move pearl up front side of left leg up to left pelvis, across solar

Sides　　　　　Front　　　　　Back

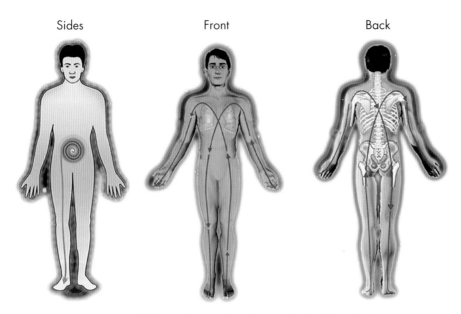

Fig. 6.18. Fusion of the Eight Psychic Channels—Sealing the Aura

plexus to right collarbone, down inside of right arm and fingers, up outside of right arm, over crown, down outside of left arm and fingers, inside of left arm to left collarbone, across chest, solar plexus, and abdomen to right hip.

6. Move flattened pearl down, covering right front leg and up backside of right leg to right buttock, across to left scapula, down inside of left arm, around left hand, up outside of left arm, over crown, down outside of right arm, up right inner arm to left scapula, across to right buttock, down left back leg to left toes. Draw pearl up left front leg to left hip to navel.

7. Collect energy at navel and do Chi Self-Massage.

ADVANCED FUSIONS
(ENERGY AND SPIRIT BODIES PRACTICES)

As noted in chapter 4, there are four spiritual creatures at the heart of Chinese mythology, each guarding a direction on the compass. Each creature has a corresponding season, color, element, and virtue. Further, each corresponds to a quadrant in the sky, with each quadrant containing seven star constellations (also called moon stations or moon lodges). There is a fifth direction—the center, representing China itself—which carries its own constellation.

From the south we receive warmth, heat, and vitality. The symbolic animal of the south is the red pheasant, which represents beauty and goodness. Portrayed with radiant feathers and an enchanting song, the red bird watches over the times of good fortune. It corresponds to summer, red, fire, and knowledge.

From the north come cold, snow, and darkness. North's symbolic animal is the black tortoise or turtle, which represents long life and endurance. Always listening, "when it becomes one thousand years old, the tortoise is able to speak the language of humans."

The direction east corresponds to springtime, green color, and the wood element, signifying new growth. East's symbolic animal is the green dragon, which represents majesty and magnificence.

The direction west corresponds to autumn and snowy mountains; it is associated with the metal element. West's symbolic animal is the white tiger, which exemplifies bravery and strength. To the Chinese the tiger was the king of all animals and lord of the mountains, and the tiger-jade ornament was especially reserved for commanders of armies. The male tiger was, among other things, the god of war, and in this capacity it not only assisted the armies of the emperors but also fought the demons that threatened the dead in their graves.

The yellow phoenix is the guardian of the center, the earth element, able to transform and bring new life from the ashes and dead matter. It has the power of both faith and acceptance.

The advanced Fusion practice that follows connects the physical, energy, and spirit bodies of the practitioner with the five sacred animals and their corresponding planets as well as with the Eight Immortals, or eight forces of nature, for superior levels of protection (see fig. 6.19).

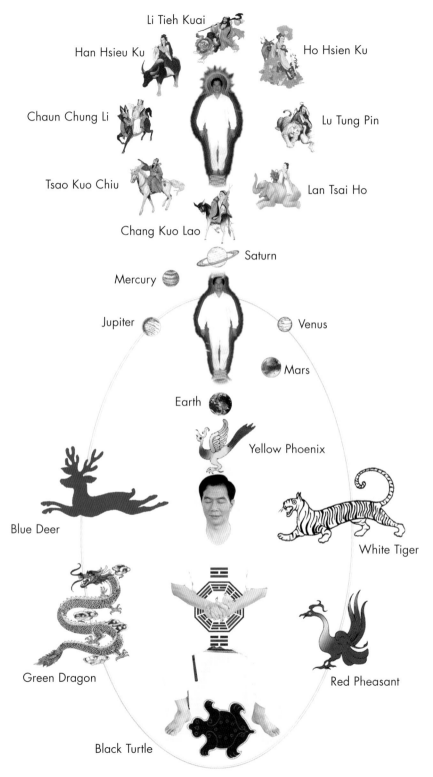

Fig. 6.19. Tri-location (animals, planets, and Eight Immortals) with nine bodies (physical, energy, and spirit bodies)

Simplified Tri-Location (Animals, Planets, and Immortals) with Nine Bodies (Physical, Energy, and Spirit Bodies)

1. Fuse energies at crown with six pakuas, forming brilliant pearl.

2. Bring pearl down to perineum and circulate in orbit.

3. Activate cranial pump by pressing tongue to lower teeth against palate, clench teeth, tilt chin back, pulling senses upward to crown, pulsating it.

4. Activate sacral pump, inhale and pull pearl from perineum to sacrum, up to T11, C7, base of skull, and crown, feeling pulsating wave extend out from crown. Exhale, feeling strong sensation of a shiny light (pearl) emerge from crown.

5. Extend pearl upward (3–6 feet), using your senses as a wireless control, moving pearl up and down, creating energy body above your crown, moving pearl 1 foot each time, to body height (see fig. 6.19 on previous page).

6. Relax senses to expand pearl, shaping it into your body shape (head, body, hands, and legs) to carve face (eyes, ears, nose, mouth). Form energy body cauldron, gender, name, and voice.

7. Form another pearl, activating cranial and sacral pumps, then exhale, guide light forcefully through crown to energy body's perineum to open its Microcosmic Orbit.

8. Spiral kidney essence to kidney collection point and feel blue light form blue virgin child and antlered deer (earth force) behind (north) physical body, connecting above with Mercury behind energy body. Breathe out black light of gentleness, forming black turtle below physical body.

9. Spiral heart essence to heart collection point and feel red light form red virgin child and red pheasant (earth force). Breathe out red light of joy, forming red pheasant in front (south) of physical body, connecting above with Mars in front of energy body.

10. Spiral liver essence to liver collection point and feel green light

form green virgin child and dragon (earth force). Breathe out green light of kindness, forming a green dragon right (east) of physical body, connecting with Jupiter right of energy body.

11. Spiral lung essence to lung collection point and feel white light form white virgin child and tiger (earth force). Breathe out white light of courage forming a white tiger left (west) of physical body connecting with Venus left of energy body.

12. Spiral spleen essence to spleen collection point and feel yellow light form yellow virgin child and phoenix (earth force). Breathe out yellow light of fairness forming a yellow phoenix above physical body, connecting with Saturn of energy body.

13. Form protective outer ring around organs with virgin children and power animals, then form protective ring and fiery dome around physical body with earth force animals in the north, south, east, west, below, and above, interconnecting with planets.

14. Form (blue and gold) compassion pearl at heart and move to cauldron in Microcosmic Orbit to energy body.

15. Exhale and send pearl to energy body heart, then exhale again and send it above energy body crown, forming spirit body.

16. Relax senses to expand pearl, shaping it into your spirit body shape (head, body, hands, and legs) carving face (eyes, ears, nose, mouth). Form spirit body cauldron, gender, and voice.

17. Run Microcosmic Orbits in physical and energy bodies then transfer light from energy body into spirit body. Do all three Microcosmic Orbits together (1 channel).

18. Extend Thrusting and Belt Channels to spirit body. Reset protective animals around physical body (black turtle below, blue deer behind, green dragon right, red pheasant front, white tiger left, and yellow phoenix above); reset planets around energy body (Earth below, Saturn above, Mars front, Mercury behind, Venus left, and Jupiter right).

19. Then, to protect the spirit body, place the Eight Immortals around it. Lu Tung Pin: Wise sage (west and Venus), tiger with sword

(yin metal, lake, and early winter); Ho Hsien Ku: Female ascetic (southwest and Saturn), deer and lotus blossom (yin earth, earth, and late summer); Lan Tsai Ho: Carnival minstrel (northwest and Neptune), elephant and flowers (yang metal, heaven, and late fall); Li Tieh Kuai: Lame beggar (south and Mars), chimera carrying a crutch (yin fire, fire, and summer); Chang Kuo Lao: Mountain recluse (north and Mercury), spirit horse and feather (yang water and winter); Han Hsieu Ku: Mountain sage (southeast and Pluto), buffalo and magic flute (yin wood, wind, and late spring); Chaun Chung Li: Army general (east and Jupiter), lion and feather fan (yang, wood/thunder, and early spring); Tsao Kuo Chiu: Mountain hermit (northeast and Uranus), spirit dragon and castanets (yang earth, mountain, and early fall).

20. Run channels (Functional, Governor, Thrusting, Belt, Bridge, and Regulator) in all three bodies connecting to North Star.

21. Select Three Different Locations: Shoot pearl into cosmos, draw down green light (3 times) at each location, forming three bodies, cleansing them, blue light washing them off, then violet light energizing them with understanding, knowledge, and wisdom, while focusing on each location.

Kan and Li Alchemy

Through Kan and Li, the Inner Sexual Alchemy of water and fire, you reunite with the Primordial Force. The heart stores part of the Primordial Force (Yuan Shen). The sexual organ also stores part of the Primordial Force. When these two combine together, they form a more complete force. The Kan and Li process establishes a powerful "steaming" effect in the tan tien cauldron at the level of the navel center. This is used to cleanse, purify, and strengthen the organs and brain to better attract the Primordial Force. Our spiritual fetus is established in the tan tien.

The equinoxes and solstices that mark the changes of the seasons provide special opportunities to get a boost of energy in these Kan and Li practices. The vernal equinox at the beginning of springtime is when the yin and yang energies are balanced between the cold water energy of winter and the hot fire energy of summer. The light of day is balanced with the darkness of night. As the cold of winter yin moves to the heat of summer yang, the earth opens its energy of the warm, moist growing power in abundance. It is a great opportunity to be open and interact with it to receive the perfectly balanced quality of water and fire energy. Humans can make use of this special offering of the Primordial Force from the earth for Inner Alchemy. This is a special time to get a huge boost of the earth's Primordial Chi.

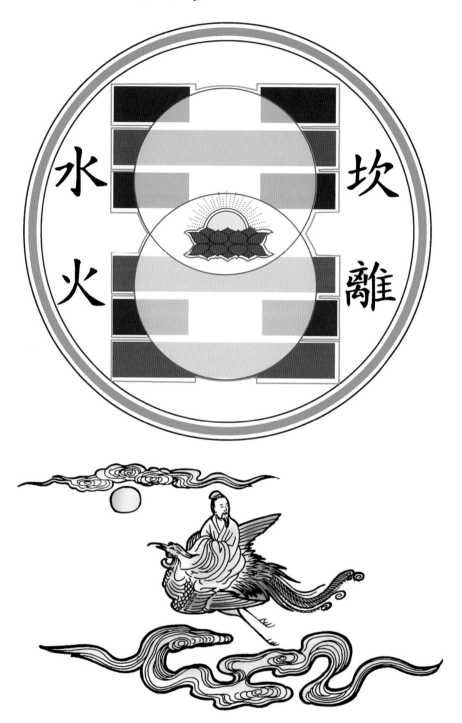

Fig. 7.1. Symbols for Kan and Li: Coupling of water and fire

LESSER KAN AND LI: TAOIST INTERNAL SEXUAL PRACTICE

Fusion practices seal off body (energy) for Kan and Li (internal energy maps). Kan and Li practices manage the polarity in the physical plane (water and fire). They are based on the Taoist theory of energy resonance fields (breathing in–breathing out) from the Wu Chi to the human. The Lesser Kan and Li practice involves the three forces: yin, yang, and neutral (center–stillness). In the act of rising and falling, there is a point that is neither rising nor falling (neutral part), which is a third channel that has no polarity. In the Tai Chi symbol there is a point or surface where both forces meet; this line (surface or point) is the neutral line. When you slow your mind, that becomes real or valid. The problem is the ego or false mind does not want to recognize it because when this appears the ego loses its identity or substance (polarity).

Alchemy is reversing the creation cycle from physical to emotional (energy) to the spiritual level on a conscious level going back to the Wu Chi (original force) through Later Heaven then Early Heaven vortexes. The main channels are: Functional (front–yin), Governor (back–yang), Core or Middle (central–neutral), Belt, Bridge (front arm and back leg) and Regulator Channels. The Middle Thrusting Channel is the core (neutral) channel of the body. The middle path, the Way of the Tao, is the core channel. The lower tan tien is the middle point of the core channel in relationship to the physical body length. Lesser Kan and Li utilizes the emotional and sexual energy to steam or transfer the energy. Then the key is that it connects back to the core channel or point, which connects us directly with the Wu Chi through all the vortexes, directly back to the source.

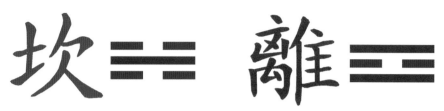

Kan: yang within yin   Li: yin within yang

Fig. 7.2. Kan and Li expressed as Chinese characters and I Ching trigrams

THE CHARACTERISTICS OF KAN AND LI

KAN	LI
Water	Fire
Yang within yin	Yin within yang
Sexual energy	Compassionate energy
Lead, true sense, endurance, stamina	Mercury, spiritual essence, virtue
Lady of the Kan in the Moon	Maiden of the Li in the Sun
North, Moon	South, Sun
White tiger	Green dragon
Female	Male
Kidney	Heart
Saliva	Chi
Semen, sperm	Blood, menstruation
Black	Red
Self	Other
True sense mixed with arbitrary feeling	Spiritual essences are adulterated with temper

The Lesser Enlightenment of Kan and Li practice combines the compassion of the heart energies (yang/fire) with sexual energies originating in the kidneys (yin/water) to form the soul, or energy, body. Practice of the Chinese formula Siaow Kan Li (yin and yang mixed) uses darkness technology to literally "steam" the sexual energy (ching) into life-force energy (chi) by reversing the location of yin and yang power. This inversion places the heat of the bodily fire from the heart center beneath the coolness of the bodily water generated by the sexual energy of the perineum, thereby activating the liberation of transformed sexual energy.

The key in Kan and Li practice is to combine the wood (+, −) and fire (+, +) with triple yang (positive) and one yin as the wood burns creating the fire; then combine water (−, −) and metal (−, +) with triple yin (negative) and one yang as the metal cauldron holds the water so it can steam the internal body. Yang (fire and wood) descends and yin (water and metal) ascends. By reversing the flow to the cauldron in the core channels, the neutral force ascends with three forces; the steam is the neutral force, which bathes all the organs.

Darkness technology has been a key element of Taoist practice— and of all Inner Alchemy traditions—throughout the ages. A total darkness environment stimulates the pineal gland to release DMT into the brain. The darkness actualizes successively higher states of consciousness, correlating with the accumulation of psychedelic chemicals in the brain. In the darkness, mind and soul begin to wander freely in the vast realms of psychic and spiritual experience. Death is no longer to be feared, because life beyond the physical body is known through direct experience. The birth of the soul is not a metaphor. It is an actual process of converting energy into a subtle body. Developing the soul body is the preparation for the growth of the immortal spirit body in the practice of the Greater Enlightenment of Kan and Li.

Simplified Lesser Kan and Li Practice

1. Smile down to kidneys, listening and feeling the kidneys' gentleness and coolness, then separate the kidney cold energy from the adrenal hot energy on top of kidneys.

2. Be aware of perineum and sexual energy. Draw down cold kidney energy (melting glacier) into water at perineum.

3. Be aware of heart and feel heart soften with the radiance of appreciation combined with ultraviolet/infrared red light and good virtues creating a compassion fire.

4. Collect hot energy of adrenals at T11 on spine and draw it up to crown, then down Middle Thrusting Channel to heart, combining with the compassion energies of heart, adrenals, and thymus at heart collection point, with mindful gentleness.

5. Create a cauldron at navel. Divide your attention with hot and cold energies at heart and perineum collection points.

6. Bring hot energy (cup of fire) down left red Thrusting Channel to perineum and cold energy (cup of water) up right blue Thrusting Channel to solar plexus without spilling any energy.

7. Move hot and cold energies into Middle Thrusting Channel and couple them at navel by exhaling, then inhaling, using the fire below as the stove boiling and steaming the water in cauldron.

8. Establish cauldron heartbeat, allowing the kidneys to pulse simultaneously with heart, pulling up sexual energy, then with the earth, and the sense automatic pulsation.

☉ Steaming Five Vital Organs and Endocrine Glands

1. Stir cauldron, mentally rocking spine, raising colored steam or vapor to each vital organ, then to all at the same time (3 times) (see fig. 7.3).

2. Smile into kidneys, gently directing blue steam into them, removing negative, sick energy with tiny blue flowers blossoming.

3. Smile into liver, gently directing green steam into it, removing negative, sick energy with tiny green flowers blossoming.

4. Smile into spleen, gently directing yellow steam into it, removing negative, sick energy with tiny yellow flowers blossoming.

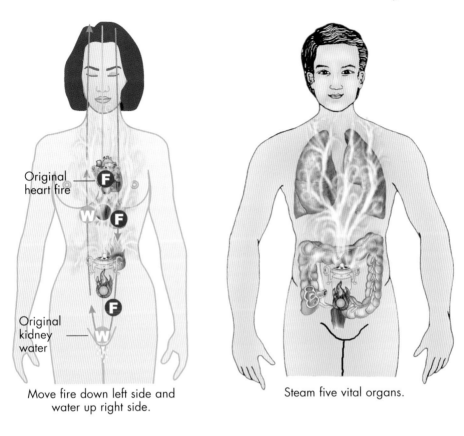

Move fire down left side and
water up right side.

Steam five vital organs.

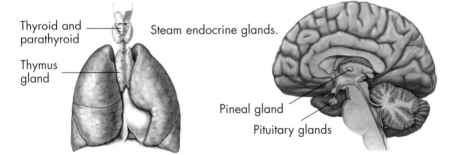

Steam endocrine glands.

Fig. 7.3. Coupling at the navel and steaming organs
and endocrine glands

5. Smile into heart, gently directing red steam into it, removing negative, sick energy with tiny red roses blossoming.

6. Smile into lungs, gently directing white steam into them, removing negative, sick energy with tiny white lilies blossoming.

7. Stir cauldron, mentally rocking spine, raising colored steam, mist, and vapor to each endocrine gland, then to all at same time.

8. Smile into thymus, thyroid, parathyroid, and salivary glands, gently directing purple steam into them, removing negative, sick energy with tiny purple violets blossoming with your breath.

9. Smile (eyes up to mid-eye) into hypothymus, pituitary, pineal, and thalamus glands, gently directing purple steam into them, removing negative, sick energy with tiny violets blossoming.

10. Smile into adrenal glands and gonads, directing purple steam into them, removing negative, sick energy with tiny violets blossoming.

☷ Steaming Spine, Lymph, Nerves

1. Exhale and push cauldron to Ming Men and stir cauldron, mentally rocking spine, raising white steam or vapor through the spinal, lymphatic, and nervous systems, then all at same time (see fig. 7.4).

2. Smile into spine; gently breathe white steam up and down spine into skull, arm, and leg bones, removing negative, sick energy with tiny white lilies blossoming, regenerating spinal cord.

3. Smile into lymph nodes and vessels; gently breathe white steam up and down pathways into chest, navel area, neck, armpits, and legs, removing negative, sick energy with tiny white lilies blossoming, cleaning out and regenerating lymphatic system.

4. Smile through spinal cord into nervous system; gently breathe white steam up and down pathways into spine, neck, head, chest, navel, arms, hands, legs, and feet, removing negative, sick energy with tiny white lilies blossoming. Let the steam clean, repair, and regenerate nervous system.

5. Repeat process with spinal, lymphatic, and nervous systems all at same time through whole body using breath in and out.

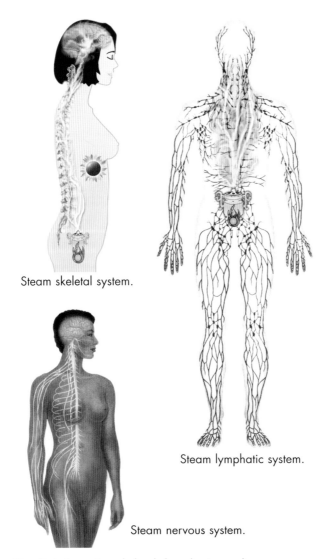

Steam skeletal system.

Steam lymphatic system.

Steam nervous system.

Fig. 7.4. Steaming skeletal, lymphatic, and nervous systems

☯ Steaming Twelve Channels

1. Stir cauldron, mentally rocking spine, raising white steam through Lung and Large Intestine channels. Hold Lung point on inside thumb edge with index finger. Breathe steam around lungs, down

inside of arms to index fingers through Lung channel. Hold thumb edge on outside index finger Lung point. Breathe white steam up outside of arms to lungs through Large Intestine channel.

2. Stir cauldron, mentally rocking spine, raising yellow steam through Stomach and Spleen channels. Hold Lung point. Breathe yellow steam from face down through stomach and legs to outside second toe (Stomach meridian) through Stomach channel. Breathe steam from inside big toe up inside legs through Spleen channel and heart to tongue (Spleen meridian).

3. Stir cauldron, mentally rocking spine, raising red steam through Heart and Small Intestine channels. Hold Heart point on pinky fingernail with thumb edge. Breathe steam around heart, down inside of arms to pinky fingers through Heart channel. Breathe red steam up outside of arms to shoulders, neck, stomach, around Small Intestine channel.

4. Stir cauldron, mentally rocking spine, raising blue steam through Urinary Bladder and Kidney channels. Hold Lung point. Breathe blue steam from bladder up over head, down back and legs to outside baby toe (Urinary Bladder meridian) through Bladder channel. Breathe blue steam from back of baby toe up inside legs to coccyx and Kidney channel (Kidney meridian).

5. Stir cauldron, mentally rocking spine, raising purple steam through Pericardium and Triple Warmer channels. Hold middle fingertips with thumbs and breathe purple steam around pericardium, down inside of arms to middle fingers through Pericardium channel. Breathe purple steam up outside arms to face, down to lower abdomen, the Triple Warmer channel.

6. Stir cauldron, mentally rocking spine, raising green steam through Gall Bladder and Liver channels. Hold Lung point and breathe green steam from face down through gallbladder and outside legs to outside fourth toe through Gall Bladder channel. Breathe steam from outside big toe up inside legs through groin and liver to face (Liver meridian) through Liver channel.

🜂 Body Pulsing and Inner Eye

1. Mentally allow heart rate to decrease and direct red steam to aorta and vena cava, feeling pulse increase to navel, groin, ankles, neck, temples, skull, armpits, inside elbows, and wrists, then amplify pulse, synchronizing pulses with North Star (see fig. 7.5).

2. Inner eye: junction between stove and cauldron forms an eye (point of light). Use it to slowly observe whole inner body.

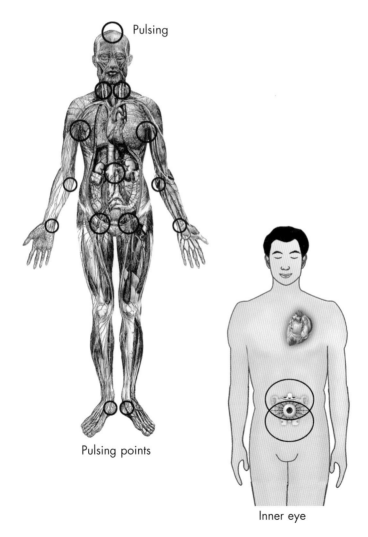

Pulsing

Pulsing points

Inner eye

Fig. 7.5. Pulsing and Inner Eye

⟳ Self-Intercourse Practice

1. Concentrate on sexual organs and pineal gland with pulsation.
2. Do power lock (3 times), drawing sexual energy up into pineal gland in Crystal Room. Use thrusts, creating orgasmic energy.
3. Draw orgasmic energy down from pineal gland to perineum through Middle Channel, compressing it in navel cauldron, expanding it out to all organs. When orgasmic energy peaks in cauldron, it creates Immortal Fetus in liver collection point (see fig. 7.6).

⟳ Turning the Wheel and Closing Practice

1. Form sexual energy pool at perineum. Looking straight ahead with eyes closed, form a mental clock. Look down into pool (6:00), drawing sexual energy up into spine with steam (see fig. 7.6).
2. Look up to the right (3:00), drawing sexual energy to T11.
3. Look up to crown (12:00), drawing energy to pineal with eyes.

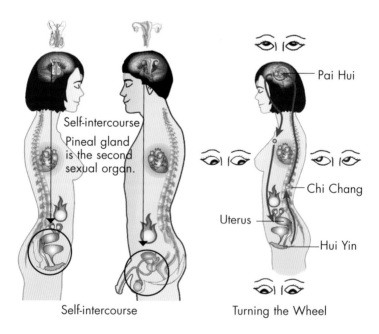

Fig. 7.6. Self-Intercourse and Turning the Wheel

4. Look down to left (9:00), draw energy down to navel cauldron.

5. Do 36 to 360 revolutions, and in time it moves independently.

GREATER KAN AND LI: SUN, MOON, AND PLANETS ALCHEMY

Greater Kan and Li Inner Alchemy practice is a secret for enlightenment in which you further reunite with the Primordial Force. Another cauldron is established in the solar plexus center to draw on the yin and yang forces of the sun, moon, and planets to further amplify the processes begun in the lower cauldron. The summer solstice marks the longest day of the year when the sun is at the highest point of its arc in our sky. All living things, the plants, flowers, and trees expand to draw on the fullness of this power of the sun. This is a great time to draw in the missing Primordial Force of the sun when we work in the cauldron at the solar plexus.

This formula comprises the Taoist Ta Kan Li (Dah Kan Li) practice. It uses the same energy relationship of yin and yang inversion but increases to an extraordinary degree the amount of energy that may be drawn up into the body. At this stage, the mixing, transforming, and harmonizing of energy takes place in the solar plexus. The increasing amplitude of power is due to the fact that the formula not only draws yin and yang energy from within the body but also draws the power directly from Heaven and Earth or ground (yang and yin, respectively), and adds the elemental powers to those of one's own body. In fact, power can be drawn from any energy source, such as the moon, wood, earth, flowers, animals, light, and so on. The formula consists of:

- Moving the stove and changing the cauldron
- Greater water and fire mixture (self-intercourse)
- Greater transformation of sexual power into the higher level

- Gathering the outer and inner alchemical agents to restore the generative force and invigorate the brain
- Cultivating the body and soul
- Beginning the refining of the sexual power (generative force, vital force, Ching Chi)
- Absorbing Mother Earth (yin) power and Father Heaven (yang) power
- Mixing with sperm and ovary power (body) and soul
- Raising the soul
- Retaining the positive, generative (creative) force, and keeping it from draining away
- Gradually doing away with food, and depending on self-sufficiency and Primordial Force
- Giving birth to the spirit
- Transferring good virtues and chi energy channels into the spiritual body
- Practicing to overcome death
- Opening the crown
- Space travelling

Building on the Lesser Kan and Li formulas for the development of the soul body, the Greater Kan and Li formulas create the immortal spirit body. Used by Taoist masters for thousands of years, these exercises are for advanced students of Taoist Inner Alchemy and mark the beginning of the path to immortality.

Greater Kan and Li reveals how to use Taoist Inner Alchemy to harness the energies of sun, moon, earth, North Star, and Big Dipper, and transform them to feed the soul body and begin development of the immortal spirit body. They explain how to reverse yin and yang power through energetic work at the solar plexus, thereby activating the liberation of transformed sexual energy. They explore how to open the heart center and how to connect astral energy with the energies of animals, children, and plants to grow the Immortal Fetus, or spirit body.

Simplified Greater Kan and Li Practice

1. Squat, gather earth blue energy rising and swallow with saliva; stand and gather heavenly energy at crown and cosmic golden energy at mid-eye.

2. Form pearl at Crystal Room with six pakuas and shoot it six body lengths out at mid-eye (human plane) (see fig. 7.7 on page 300), then six body lengths down to perineum into earth plane, then out crown (heavenly plane,) then run Microcosmic Orbit, Thrusting Channels, and Belt Channels through planes.

3. Feel anchor support as you rock spine and reverse hot and cold energies from perineum and Crystal Room to navel and heart, coupling at solar plexus cauldron by exhaling, then inhale.

4. Steam kidneys, liver, spleen, heart, and lungs, then endocrine glands and lymphatic, spinal, and nervous systems with colors and blooming tiny flowers and fragrances, then through all twelve channels.

5. Do bellows breathing to activate all pulses to North Star.

6. Adjust outer seasonal temperatures in cauldron with yang tiger in sky and water and yin dragon in sky and water.

7. Connect with vital organs' inner animal and virgin child with blue waterfall, red volcano, green forest, white mountain, and yellow desert, via pure energy in vital organs.

8. Shoot pearl into the earth for your animal soul guides.

9. Activate self-intercourse with thrusting and pulsation techniques to give birth to Immortal Fetus (soul/spirit) by marrying the light, moving up to all organs, to crown, and above head.

10. Form outer energy and spirit bodies connecting to North Star and personal star, going to light, drawing energy to bodies.

11. Astral flight: Focus on third eyes of three bodies and push orgasmic energy up spine and out and physical third eye with Orgasmic Upward Draw technique (9–18 times) focusing on vertical projection out of forehead.

12. Turning the Wheel—do Sun, Moon, Tree, and Star practices. (See "Simplified Sun, Moon, Tree, Star Practices" on page 185.)

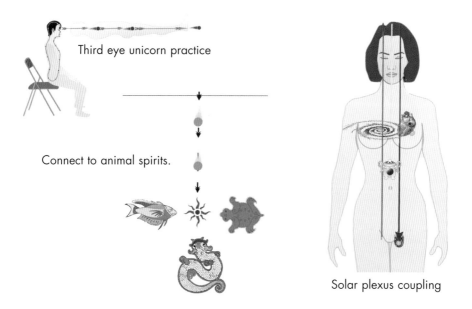

Third eye unicorn practice

Connect to animal spirits.

Solar plexus coupling

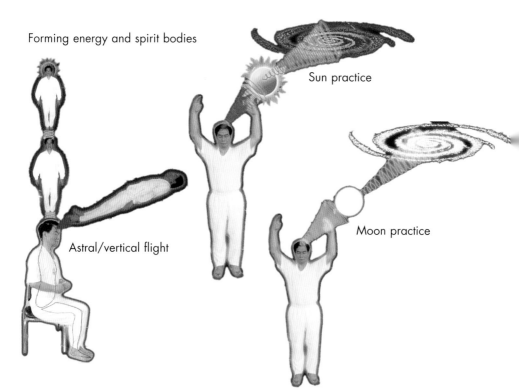

Forming energy and spirit bodies

Sun practice

Astral/vertical flight

Moon practice

Fig. 7.7. Greater Kan and Li Practice

GREATEST KAN AND LI:
PLANET, STAR, AND SOUL ALCHEMY

The Greatest Kan and Li practices offer the possibility of reuniting with the Internal Alchemy Primordial Force still more. You establish another cauldron in the heart center and expand the body to become a cosmic being, billions of light years from head to toe: an immense being of the universe whose Crystal Palace is the North Star with constellations and planets for vital Internal Alchemy organs. Be this being that beams down its exquisite rays to one cell of its being, the human on planet Earth meditating up to the stars.

Cosmic consciousness opens the three Internal Alchemy tan tiens to receive Primordial Force from their heavenly counterpart. By manifesting the intention to connect the relevant heavenly bodies to the appropriate parts of our body, we attract the cosmic primordial forces needed for our Internal Alchemy to further develop our energy (soul) body and spirit body. This more refined alchemy in the heart cauldron enhances and furthers the steaming processes of the energies of water and fire, yin and yang, begun in the lower cauldrons.

The autumnal equinox at the beginning of the fall season is when the yin and yang energies are balanced between the hot fire energy of summer and the cold water energy of winter. The days and nights are balanced as the days become shorter. As the heat of summer yang moves to the cold of winter yin, it's a good time to get extra benefit in the Greatest Kan and Li practice of drawing the missing heavenly Primordial Force into the body. In resonance with the tendency of the weather, the cells of the body are contracting and drawing inward from the cool dry weather after the expanding heat of the summer.

The soul body is yin energy, and the spiritual body is yang energy. The soul body serves as an earth cable and absorbs the yang energy from the heavenly "wire" down to the human body. It also absorbs the earth energy to balance the yang energy absorbed from the heavenly (spirit) body. This Internal Alchemy formula is yin and yang power mixed at a higher energy center. It helps to reverse the aging process by reestablishing the thymus gland and increasing natural immunity. This means that healing energy is radiated from a more powerful point in the body, providing greater benefits to the physical and ethereal bodies.

The formula consists of:

- Moving the stove and changing the cauldron to the higher center
- Absorbing the solar and lunar power
- Greatest mixing, transforming, steaming, and purifying of sexual power (generative force), soul, Mother Earth, Father Heaven, solar and lunar power
- Mixing the visual power with the vital power
- Mixing (sublimating) the body, soul, and spirit

After mastering the Inner Alchemy practices of Lesser Kan and Li and Greater Kan and Li, the advanced student is now ready for the refinement of the soul and spirit made possible through the practice of the Greatest Kan and Li. Through the practice you discover the merging energy at the heart center, which leads to the birth of the immortal spirit body, uniting you with the Tao and allowing you to draw limitless energy and power from the cosmos.

 ## Simplified Greatest Kan and Li Practice

1. Empty heart (black hole) of desires, thoughts, and things.
2. Form six pakuas in Crystal Room; gather the light into a pill.
3. Form pearl at Crystal Room with six pakuas and shoot it six body lengths out at mid-eye (human plane) then six body lengths down to perineum into earth plane, then out crown (heavenly plane), then run Microcosmic Orbit, Thrusting Channels, and Belt Channels through planes.

4. Reverse hot and cold energies from perineum and throat center to navel and solar plexus, forming cauldron at heart with breath (see fig. 7.8).

5. Steam kidneys, liver, spleen, heart, and lungs, then endocrine glands and lymphatic, spinal, and nervous systems, with colors and blooming tiny flowers and fragrances, then through twelve channels.

6. Do bellows breathing, activating pulses to North Star and inner eye.

7. Draw dark cloudy color from fire and toes into heart, down through

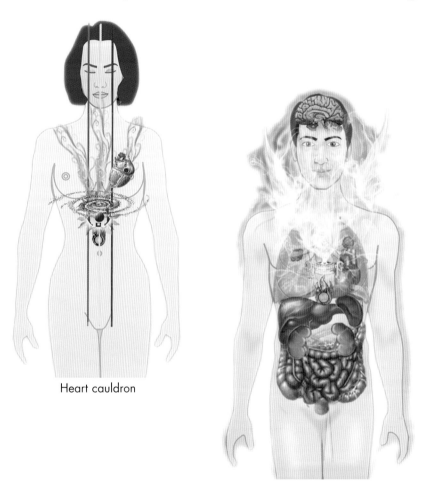

Heart cauldron

Steaming organs, channels, and body systems from the heart cauldron

Fig. 7.8. Greatest Kan and Li: steaming from the heart cauldron

the spine, doing heart's sound (haw-w-w-w-w-w), steam and empty heart, letting go of all attachments through spine and toes.

8. Align the three triangles (tan tiens at Crystal Room, heart, and sacrum) connecting with heavenly forces (10 stems) and earth forces (12 branches) (upper and lower) and spiral vortexes clockwise and counterclockwise to receive the light.

9. Pulsate and steam heart with aorta (sun), vena cava (moon), right and left atrium and ventricle (4 heart chambers), then through Regulator, Bridge, Belt, Thrusting, Functional, and Governor Channels, twelve meridians, nerves, and bones.

10. Listen to the movement of emptiness as the blood flows through inferior and superior vena cava, right atrium, left atrium, pulmonary vein, right and left ventricles, pulmonary artery, aorta, and the rest of the body.

11. Connect skull with south, north, west, and east constellations, Big Dipper's seven stars and North Star (see fig. 7.9 on facing page):

    Alcor (7–crown)

    Mizar (6–Jade Pillow)

    Alioth (5–chin)

    Megrez (4–left temple)

    Phecda (3–right temple)

    Merak (2–right ear)

    Dubhe (1–left ear)

    Polaris (Crystal Room)

12. Marry the light: See first light (dim, cloudy, small pill, holy spirit). Form pakuas at navel, crown, mid-eye, and palms, drawing and condensing light into pakuas, and spiral into cauldron forming a pearl (embryo). Close eyes and see light inside mixing with second

Fig. 7.9 (opposite). Connecting Big Dipper's seven stars and North Star with skull: Alcor (7–crown), Mizar (6–Jade Pillow), Alioth (5–chin), Megrez (4–left temple), Phecda (3–right temple), Merak (2–right ear), Dubhe (1–left ear), and Polaris (Crystal Room)

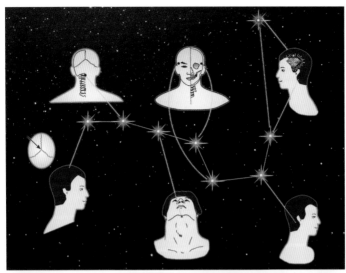

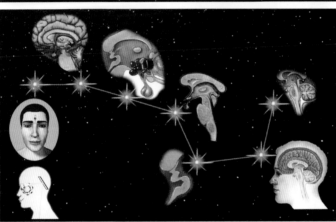

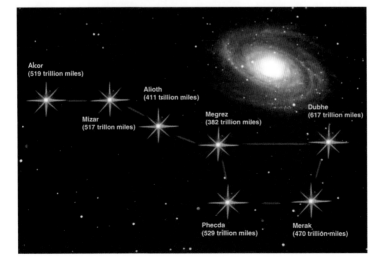

Alcor
(519 trillion miles)

Alioth
(411 trillion miles)

Mizar
(517 trillon miles)

Megrez
(382 trillion miles)

Dubhe
(617 trillion miles)

Phecda
(529 trillion miles)

Merak
(470 trillion miles)

outside light, forming red light. See a dragon (right and high sound) and tiger (left and low sound). Feel fetus (red baby) breathe and grow on its own, pulsating with you.

13. Third outside light appears; draw it down to cauldron, sealing senses and anus. Feel stirring in cauldron (pregnancy) and collect saliva. Do a slow, even, long breath, until there is no breath, and move light to nose and do self-intercourse, then orbit.

14. End the meditation with Turning the Wheel (see fig. 7.10) and do Bone Breathing practices.

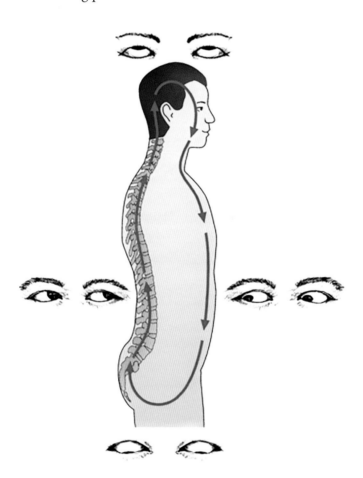

Fig. 7.10. Turning the Wheel

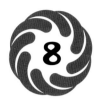

Star and Galaxy Alchemy

SEALING OF THE FIVE SENSES

Finally, we add the cauldron in the head, the upper tan tien. This cauldron is located at the mid-eyebrow point. It unifies the five shen, the five streams of personal consciousness that operate through our senses, with the five forces of the collective stellar self. The body of our stellar mind can be viewed in the four quadrants of fixed stars in the night sky, originally symbolized by heraldic animals (black turtle, red pheasant, green dragon, and white tiger). The fifth, the quintessence, is the purple pole star in the center of the sky, with the Great Bear of the Big Dipper marking the progression of the seasons as its handle rotates like the arm of a cosmic clock. These personal and stellar essences are fused in the upper tan tien at the mid-eyebrow point. This is the process of our inner sage attaining the celestial level of immortality. The pure open space connecting the three tan tien cauldrons (at the navel, heart, and mid-eyebrow) is integrated. This stabilizes the celestial axis. Profound peace and different spiritual qualities continuously manifest from this activated core and radiate sonically into our physical becoming. We hear the current of inner sound.

Our soul pattern expands its conscious destiny to include dimensions of life beyond the physical plane. This very high formula effects a transmutation of the warm current or chi into mental energy or energy of the soul. To do this, we must seal the five senses, for each one is an open gate of energy loss. In other words, power flows out from each of the sense organs unless there is an esoteric sealing of these doors of energy movement. They must release energy only when specifically called upon to convey information. Abuse of the senses leads to far more energy loss and degradation than people ordinarily realize. Each of the elements has a corresponding sense through which its elemental force may be gathered or spent. The eye corresponds to fire; the tongue to water; the left ear to metal; the right ear to wood; the nose to earth.

Sealing of the Five Senses formula consists of:

- Sealing the five thieves: ears, eyes, nose, tongue, and body
- Controlling the heart and seven emotions (pleasure, anger, love, hate, and desire)
- Uniting and transmuting the inner alchemical agent into life-preserving true vitality
- Purifying and raising the spirit; stopping the spirit from wandering outside in quest of sense data
- Eliminating decayed food and depending on undecayed food, the Primordial Force

In ancient times, the Sealing of the Five Senses involved both Taoist Inner Alchemy and physical sealing of the sensory organs to prepare the master for extended periods of astral travel and meditation. In modern times, physical sealing of the senses with wax is no longer required. However, in order to accumulate profound energy and gather cosmic light for the immortal spirit body, one must stop the energy losses that occur through the senses. The nine Inner Alchemy formulas for the

Sealing of the Five Senses practice include strengthening the senses, connecting the senses to the organs, activating the Thrusting Channels, and harnessing the energies of the Big Dipper and the North Star. These practices build upon the formulas of the Lesser, Greater, and Greatest Kan and Li, all of which reverse the polarity of fire and water in the body, placing Li (fire) energy beneath a cauldron that contains Kan (water) energy. To stop energy losses through the five senses and transmute warm chi into energy for the immortal spirit body, proper diet and eating habits are a part of this practice.

Abuse of the senses leads to energy loss and degradation. Through this practice you are shown how sealing the senses allows you to create the Crystal Room cauldron, where fire and water energy can couple to generate a superior essence used to achieve greater awareness and "steam" all the body's major organ systems. The purifying steam produced by Kan and Li practices permits gestation and nurturing of an Immortal Fetus, a spirit body that can leave the physical body to commune with the energies of the universe.

Simplified Sealing of the Five Senses Practice

Formula 1: Crystal Room Cauldron

1. Do Inner Smile and bellows breathing then activate yin fire (tiger) and yang fire (dragon). Be aware of left ear (metal force–yin fire) and right ear (wood force–yang fire). Draw two forces together into Crystal Room combining into fire force.

2. Be aware of mouth and breathe into mouth, gathering water force. Create collection points for water in mouth and fire in Crystal Room. Raise water up and lower fire down, then couple at nose tip, drawing steam to Crystal Room.

❂ *Formula 2:*
Sun and Moon Cauldron

1. Be aware of left eye (sun power) and right eye (moon power) (see fig. 8.1A).
2. Combine two powers into the nose bridge to become fire force (see fig. 8.1B). Breathe in external chi to form a chi ball in mouth.
3. Raise water and lower fire down, then couple at nose tip, drawing steam to Crystal Room.

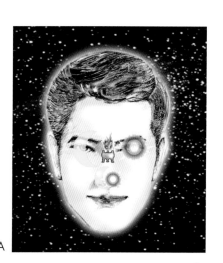 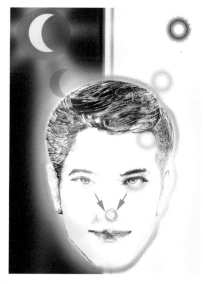

A   B

Fig. 8.1. Sealing of the Five Senses:
Sun and Moon Cauldron

❂ *Formula 3:*
True Kidney (Weaving Maiden) Cauldron

1. Raise up fire force from left kidney to left ear collection point.
2. Be aware of lower cauldron and feel fire start to warm abdomen, then steam sexual organs, transforming sexual energy into chi. Let this energy rise to right (yin–Weaving Maiden) kidney to activate the essence of sexual energy (inner yang). Raise right kidney energy to right ear collection point.

3. Let left and right ear (fire and water) couple in Crystal Room (middle of the ear). Be aware of mouth; gather water force into a chi ball and couple with fire at nose (earth).

☸ Formula 4:
Building Aura Fields

1. Open Thrusting Channels and activate sexual energy.
2. Turning the Wheel: Move energy up spine to T11, then down to lower tan tien, up spine to C7, then down to solar plexus and up spine to brain, then down to heart.
3. Build the aura around the body (see fig. 8.2): Breathe red mist into heart, then exhale gray colors from heart; send out red mist to create an aura around body. Breathe yellow mist into spleen, then exhale gray colors from spleen, sending yellow mist to nose;

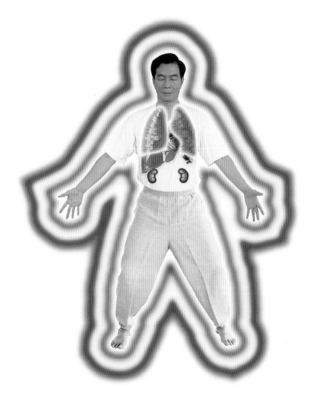

Fig. 8.2. Sealing of the Five Senses: Building Aura Fields

from mouth breathe out yellow mist to create an aura. Breathe white mist into lungs and breathe out gray colors from lungs, then send white mist to nose; from nose breathe out white mist to create an aura. Breathe blue mist into kidneys, then breathe out gray colors from kidneys, sending blue mist to ears; from ears breathe out blue mist to create an aura. Breathe green mist into liver and breathe out gray colors, then from liver send green mist to eyes; from eyes breathe green mist out to create an aura around the body.

4. Be aware of entire rainbow aura radiating around you, building from each of the organs and feel it expand as you breathe.

⊘ Formula 5:
Fire (Sun) and Water/Sexual Energy (Moon) Cauldron

1. Bring sun to left eye (fire) then to bridge of nose and moon to right eye (water) then to mid-eye. Start coupling the two different energies and feel steam come out of the third eye.
2. Gather sexual energy from sexual organs, then bring it to the collection point in mouth, then the steam produced from sun and moon becomes fire for coupling at the tip of nose.
3. Bring fire energy down to upper lip and water energy from mouth to bridge of the nose and start coupling at tip of nose, feeling suction. Let fire cool and bring it down to lower tan tien.

⊘ Formula 6:
Four Protection Forces

1. Harmonizing four forces at earth center to be nourished, strengthened, and sealed: eyes (green dragon–east–wood) are not seeing and eternal soul stays in liver, turning eye power inward. Ears (blue tortoise–north–water) are not hearing, and sexual essence stays in

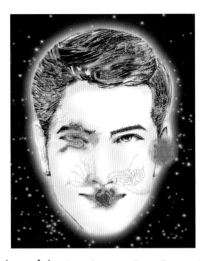

Fig. 8.3. Sealing of the Fire Senses: Four Protection Forces

kidneys, then turn ears inward. Tongue (red pheasant–south–fire) is not speaking and spirit stays in heart, then turn tongue power inward. Nose (white tiger–west–metal) is not smelling and corporeal soul stays in lungs. Then regulate breath inward (see fig. 8.3).

2. Send out the pill (pearl) to connect with Big Dipper, then connect stars to left and right temples, left and right mastoid, chin, base of skull and crown, then North Star to Crystal Room.

3. See Big Dipper full of violet light and violet light now pouring into crown. Draw sun to left eye (fire), to bridge of nose, and moon to right eye (water), to mid-eye, then start coupling the two different energies and steam will come out the third eye.

4. Rise up fire force from left (true) kidney to left ear collection point. Let this energy rise to right (yin–Weaving Maiden) kidney to activate the stored essence of sexual energy (inner yang) then let right kidney energy rise to right ear (collection point). Let left and right ear (fire and water) couple in Crystal Room (middle of the ear).

5. Bring sexual energy up to pineal gland and allow it to drip down to mouth, then mix it with saliva and fill mouth with sexual energy.

Draw fire energy down from Crystal Room to upper lip and water energy up from mouth to the bridge of nose, then couple at tip of the nose.

6. Be aware of ears, feeling blue energy turning into a tortoise in each ear to seal and protect ears. Be aware of nose, feeling white energy turning into white tiger in nose to seal and protect nose. Be aware of eyes, feeling green energy turning into green dragons in eyes to seal and protect eyes. Be aware of tongue, feeling red energy turning into red pheasant in mouth protecting tongue.

7. Draw green (wood) energy of eyes down to tongue (fire) and combine them to create one fire energy, then send fire to Crystal Room. Draw white (metal) energy from nose over to ears (water) and combine them to create one water energy. Send water to Crystal Room; then couple water and fire in Crystal Room. Slowly simmer for a long time, emptying your mind into the lower tan tien anytime thoughts arise. Feel the stillness of your senses. Feel how they are sealed, and slowly let the fire cool down.

❂ Formula 7: Energy and Planet Protection

1. Clean out the Thrusting Channels and activate sexual energy in lower tan tien.

2. Turn the Wheel and build the aura and send pearl to connect with Big Dipper stars, then feel violet light pouring into your crown and connect North Star to Crystal Room.

3. Wash the whole body and bone marrow with violet light.

4. Activate kidneys with ears and collection points, coupling fire and water in Crystal Room, then activate sun and moon with eyes and collection points, coupling fire and water at nose tip.

5. Be aware of all three couplings simultaneously, then Crystal Room steam forms a pearl and opens up third eye.

6. Send liver energy out to draw in green planet, Jupiter, sealing and

protecting your eyes. Send heart energy out to draw in red planet, Mars, sealing and protecting your tongue (mouth). Bring eyes to mouth, combining eyes and tongue, creating fire energy, drawing it up to Crystal Room.

7. Send kidney energy out to draw in blue planet, Mercury, sealing and protecting your ears. Send lung energy out to draw in white planet, Venus, sealing and protecting your nose. Bring ears to nose, combining them, creating water energy, and draw it up to Crystal Room.

8. Start coupling fire and water at Crystal Room, letting all thoughts go, sending them to lower tan tien.

❷ Formula 8: Big Dipper Cauldron

1. Do bellows breathing, connecting lower tan tien, then build aura with mist. Send out pearl to connect your personal star to Big Dipper and look for the light.

2. Draw Big Dipper in, connect to your head (left and right temples), right mastoid, chin, base of skull, and crown, and connect North Star to Crystal Room. See and feel Big Dipper pouring out violet light down into your crown then your whole body. Wash your body in violet light deep into your bone marrow and feel your body filled and overflowing with the violet light, creating an aura around your body.

3. Be aware of coupling at mid-eyebrow, Crystal Room, and tip of nose, and feel aura move in and out with your breath, and let your fire cool down.

❷ Formula 9: Connecting the Four Constellations

1. Do bellows breathing, connecting with lower tan tien, then expand mind to east constellations (liver and wood), south constellations

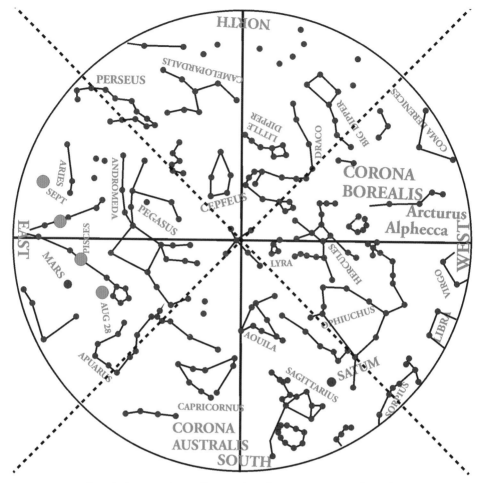

Fig. 8.4. Four Constellations (north, east, west, and south)

(heart and fire), west constellations (lungs and metal), and north constellations (kidneys and water), using the Crystal Room as the center point (see fig. 8.3 on page 316).

2. Combine south constellation (fire) and east constellation (wood), creating one fire energy. Combine north constellation (water) and west constellation (metal), creating one water energy. Then couple them at Crystal Room, feeling the aura move with breath, refining all four constellations' energies.

3. Be aware of planets and animals protecting and sealing your senses

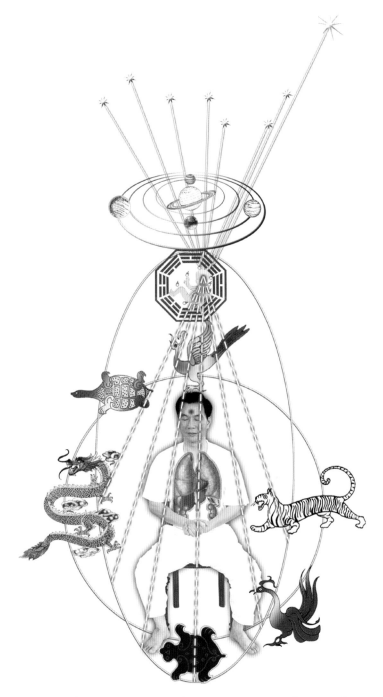

Fig. 8.5. Pearl connecting to North Star, Big Dipper, planet and animal
protection forces, and organs

(see fig. 8.4 on page 316). Shoot energy body out and make yourself very large, connecting with four constellations.

4. Start coupling constellation energies, feeling vast amounts of energy beaming down to your Crystal Room and heart, then see rainbow beams coming out from your heart around your body. Bring your awareness to lower tan tien and couple it, using this energy to heal your body and mind.

5. Slowly simmer for a long time, emptying your mind into lower tan tien. Anytime thoughts arise, feel the stillness of your senses and feel how they are sealed. Slowly let fire cool down.

6. Collect and gather the energy in the lower tan tien.

CONGRESS OF HEAVEN AND EARTH

This practice integrates the Early Heaven or formless self with the Later Heaven (Earth) physical self. The self here identifies with two dimensions that coexist and co-create: the "formless form" of our being and the "substantial form" of our becoming. These two polar dimensions of our greater self engage in cosmic sex. They couple in order to re-open the portal to their original state, or "pre-self." This pre-state or Primordial Heaven is called *Hundun*, the primal chaos-unity that preceded the "Big Bang" of the cosmic egg cracking open. The Three Treasures of Heaven, Earth, and Humanity are gathered in the three body cauldrons as Original Ching, Original Chi, and Original Shen. This three-tone harmonic chord is resonated with the fundamental or original tone of time and space.

Consciousness then stabilizes in the axial center where our true multidimensional nature can now be embodied. This is symbolized by a tonal double vortex spinning faster than the speed of light within the void of space. Into this is fused our inner sage's immortal presence, the quintessence of humanity meditating in the center of a cosmic torus (spiritual black hole). We must enter this portal to complete our journey

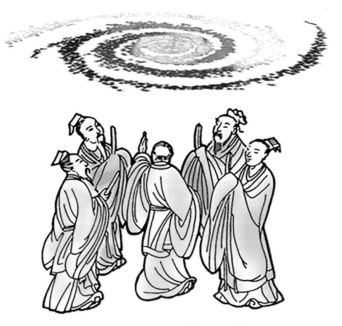

Fig. 8.6. Heaven and Earth Alchemy

of return to the origin. This formula is difficult to describe in words. It involves the incarnation of a male and a female entity within the body of the practitioner. These two entities have sexual intercourse within the body. It involves the mixing of the yin and yang powers on and about the crown of the head, being totally open to receive energy from above, and the regrowth of the pineal gland to its fullest use. When the pineal gland has developed to its fullest potential, it will serve as a compass to tell us in which direction our aspirations can be found. Taoist esotericism is a method of mastering the spirit, as described in Taoist alchemy. Without the body, the Tao cannot be attained, but with the body, truth can never be realized.

This formula consists of:

- Mingling (uniting) the body, soul, spirit with the universe
- Fully developing the positive to eradicate the negative completely
- Returning the spirit to nothingness

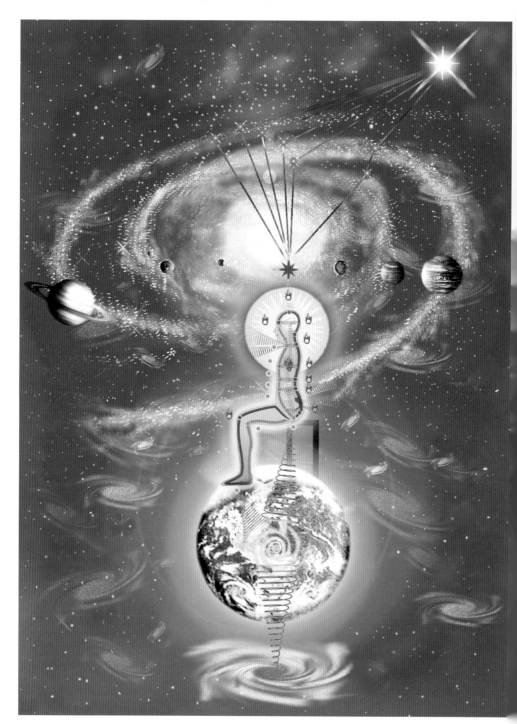

Fig. 8.7. Supreme Unknown Alchemy

REUNION OF HEAVEN AND MAN: SUPREME UNKNOWN ALCHEMY

This stage is the integration of the eight previous levels of consciousness into the experience of living simultaneously in the present moment in all dimensions, from physical linear time to spirit's eternal time. This state cannot be fully known or defined conceptually for others. Perhaps it might be conceptualized as the experience of living fully in the Wu Chi, the Supreme Unknown. This is the true achievement of the authentic or immortal self, a permanent state of grace known as Wu Wei, effortless action, or spontaneous action without acting. Creation (of the manifest) and return to formless origin seamlessly complete each other. Attainment of this ninth level is spontaneous, and it happens when the inner will of our immortal sage within has reached complete

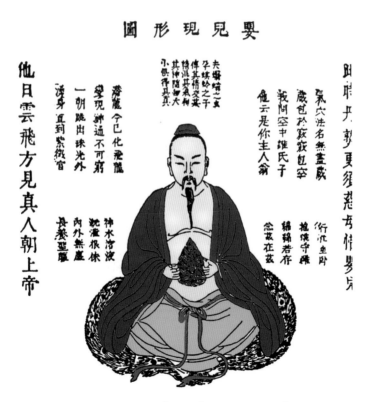

Fig. 8.8. Cosmology of Taoist Immortality

alignment with the Tao. It may occur only by direct transmission from the Tao to the mature and receptive adept.

We compare the body to a ship, and the soul to the engine and propeller of a ship. This ship carries a very precious and very large diamond, which it is assigned to transport to a very distant shore. If your ship is damaged (a sick and ill body), no matter how good the engine is, you are not going to get very far and may even sink. Thus, we advise against spiritual training unless all of the channels in the body have been properly opened and made ready to receive the 10,000 or 100,000 volts of superpower that will pour down into them. The Taoist approach, which has been passed down to us for over five thousand years, consists of many thousands of methods. The formulae and practices we describe in these books are based on such secret knowledge and the authors' own experience during more than forty years of study and of successfully teaching thousands of students.

The main goal of the Reunion of Heaven and Man Taoist practices is to overcome reincarnation and the fear of death through enlightenment of the higher level of the immortal spirit and life after death. This highest level is the immortal spirit in an immortal body. This body functions like a mobile home or space ship to the spirit and soul as it moves through the subtle planes, allowing greater power of manifestation.

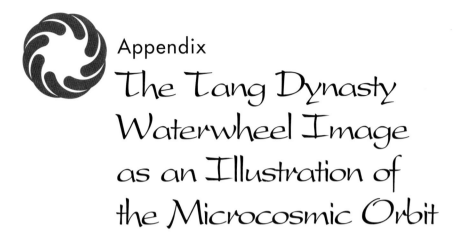

Appendix

The Tang Dynasty Waterwheel Image as an Illustration of the Microcosmic Orbit

HISTORICAL OVERVIEW

The ancient rendering illustrating the Internal Alchemy method was probably originally drawn by a highly achieved Taoist from China's Tang Dynasty period (seventh century CE). This was a golden period of Internal Alchemy, during which many Taoist and Chan Buddhist schools (mixed Tao-Buddhist teachings later known as "Zen" in Japan) and monasteries received imperial support. Many dynasties later, the drawing was discovered by a Taoist adept, who added this inscription at the bottom of the chart:

> The original chart was found hanging in the library at High Pine Mountain, where it was concealed from public view for many hundreds of years. Perhaps the diagram of the inner world hidden within our own body was too deep and mysterious for it to be well understood by the outer world. The original chart was clearly drawn and printed, so it was easily reprinted after its importance was realized. When I first saw it I decided it was too precious not to be shared with everyone. So I humbly offer again to the world that spirit.
>
> SUN TUN

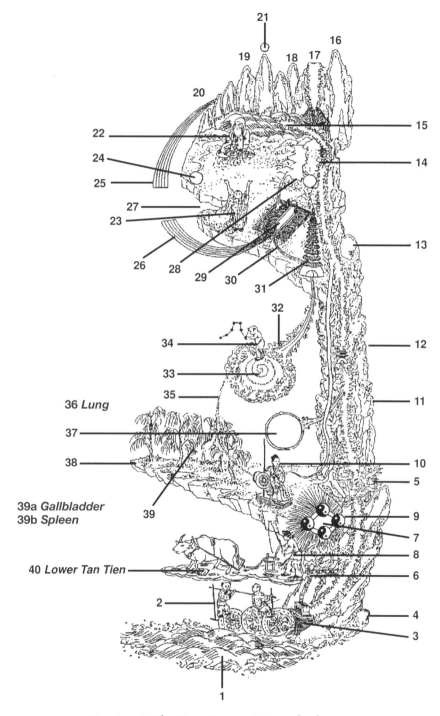

36 *Lung*

39a *Gallbladder*
39b *Spleen*

40 *Lower Tan Tien*

Fig. App.1. The Tang Dynasty Waterwheel image

In the same spirit as the internal alchemists living in ancient China, the Universal Healing Tao again offers this chart to the public, only this time we decode its strange symbols so that modern people can understand the mysterious relationship between their body, nature, and the universe. The ancient Taoist saw the human body as a microcosm of the natural world. Our physical anatomy is an inner landscape with its own rivers, forests, mountains, and lakes, which reflect their harmony with the outer landscape of the planet Earth. You can see the outline of the spine rising to the spiritual peaks within the head and brain. The drawing refers to the meridians of the Microcosmic Orbit (the small heavenly circle). This is the warm current circulation that is a central part of the Taoist alchemy. The true purpose of alchemy is the internal development, purification, and transmutation of our vital organs and sexual energy.

OUTLINE OF THE DRAWING

Sexual energy is the major ingredient of the Inner Alchemy. The key to figure App.1 is:

1. The Sea of Water (river of sexual energy), which flows downstream. To be able to make the water (sexual energy) flow upstream is the beginning of the Inner Alchemy, the higher spiritual practice.

2. The Boy and Girl at the perineum (CV 1) represent the testicles and the ovaries, or the left and right eyes. When we feel sexually aroused or feel orgasm and can simultaneously become aware of a loving feeling, we can start the inner alchemical process. By using the power of our mind and heart, along with the rolling of our eyes, to move the energy of our sexual organs, we can begin to blend the energies of sex and love, and to change their properties until they become light and begin to flow to the first gate.

3. This gate, as it is explained in the text, lies to the east at the tip of the coccyx, or the Gate of the Tail. This center is a reunion point between both kidneys. This is the first step on a ladder (GV 1) ascending to the Celestial Heights. No matter how much sexual arousal or orgasm energy we have—referred to in the text as a lake with a depth of ten thousand fathoms—this method will transform it and pump it upward.

4. The next center is the sacral hiatus (GV 2), shown as a long slab of rock with eight holes. It is also known as the Immortal Caves, which are able to receive the energies of the earth and blend them with the sexual energies.

5. The energy moves up to the House of the Two Kidneys (CV 4).

6. This alchemical process starts from the lower abdomen in the navel area (lower tan tien) as a cauldron burning with fire. The flames are cooking and transforming the sexual energy.

7. The four yin and yang symbols within one circle are moving the life force and sexual energy that has been accumulating from the Burning Cauldron in the lower tan tien. This is experienced as a warm, glowing, radiating feeling in both a vortex and centrifugal form known as chi.

8. The Buffalo corresponds to the earth energy and stubbornness and the Plow Boy symbolizes the need to cultivate the inner self before the seed (Immortal Fetus) can be planted and its fruits can be harvested or the gold coin can be minted. The earth (spleen–yellow) is the central ground of our being and the source of fundamental nourishment.

9. The four yin/yang symbols also represent the eight trigrams of the I Ching and move in harmony to manifest the physical body. The area below the kidneys, in front of the spinal cord, is also known as the True Tan Tien. When you concentrate on the right point you will feel the chi build up and rush up to the crown.

10. The Weaving Maiden, represented by the right kidney, is yin and

is the genuine water that stores the inner yang, attracting the active yang.

11. The energy moves up through the rocky vertebrae to the center at T11 (GV 6) in the middle of the spine, which is the point between the adrenal glands.

12. The energy moves up to the next center, T5 (GV 11), which is the Spirit Path in the Tower at the same level of the heart. This is seen as a vantage point from which our spirit can survey our journey before going into the Higher Spirit Path.

13. As we ascend through the rocky vertebrae, we come to C7 (GV 14), the Big Hammer, where all yang meridians are united.

14. The next gate is at the base of the skull, the Jade Pillow (GV 16).

15. Then the energy flows upward to the head, and ultimately through the crown, where it connects with the Sea of Brain Marrow.

16.–20. The energy moves to the top of the head, where the nine peaks of the mountain and their caves are located. This is Kun Lun Mountain, which is one of the sacred places in the Tao. It is the land of immortality. These peaks connect to the crown points, which have a close connection to the universal force.

21. Immortal Realm Peak, along with the pearl above it, represents the essence of the life force and sexual energy transmuted into spiritual and wisdom energy. The purpose of this transmutation is to reunite the higher self, represented by the pearl, with the spirit.

22. The wise man, Lao Tzu, is sitting in the original cavity of our spirit at mid-eyebrow (GV 24) in the Spirit Hall of the Courtyard.

23. Bodhidharma, the founder of Zen Buddhism in China, is the man holding up his hands to connect to the heavenly energy.

24. The Two Circles are the eyes, which are the Boy and Girl stepping on the waterwheel to move energy in our body.

25–26. The bands of rainbow stripes represent the Governor and the Conception Channels meeting at their exit points. The five lines in each band show that they carry the five predominantly yang and yin energies of the organs.

27. When we touch the tongue (Drawbridge) to the upper palate, these two meridians connect together and complete the circuit of chi.

28. The sweet nectar or elixir pours downward from the Dew Pond, which gives inner nutrition to the brain.

29. It reaches the brain via the Mouth Pool (GV 28), called the Mouth Crossing.

30. At this point (CV 24), we receive the fluid forming the Heavenly Pool.

31. The flow of the nectar and chi continues down the throat (Twelve-Storied Pagoda) to CV 22, or the "Heaven Rushing Out."

32. The stream of nectar flows into the Flaming Balls of Fire at the pericardium, which helps cool and irrigate the heart.

33. At the center of the heart is a Spiral of Rice Grains, which is one of the twelve symbols used in imperial decoration. The rice grains symbolize abundance. One tiny grain of rice contains the whole universe within.

34. The Divine Cowherder places the stars in the Big Dipper. This provides a guide for both the seasons and the location of the Pole Star. This also helps collect the astral power, which we learn to gather.

35. The Milky Way helps make the connection between the heart and the kidneys, harmonizing the forces of water and fire.

36. The Lung spirit (Hwa Hao) finds fullness in the empty space; then the function of the lung is completed.

37. The solar plexus is known as the middle tan tien.

38. We move down to the Outer Ring of the Forest representing the edge of the rib cage.

39. The Forest of Trees connects to the liver, the wood element.

39a. The Gall Bladder spirit (Lung Au) is called the Majestic and Bright Spirit.

39b. The Spleen spirit (Chaeng Tsai) is called the Soul Pavilion.

40. The energy finally descends back down to the lower tan tien, which includes a Boy Plowing with a Buffalo, the Burning Cauldron (6) and the moving of the four yin and yang (Tai Chi) balls (7). The flow of chi (life force) travels back down to the Sea of Water (1) to make a complete circle.

Each time the chi flows back down it becomes more refined. When we pump it up again and again, we continue to transform and refine the energy further. In this way we activate a natural process of energy recycling, which provides us with a never-ending supply of life force.

DETAILED EXPLANATION

1. We have to learn to reverse the flow of our sexual energy, which, like water, always tends to flow down and run out. Sexual energy is the most vital life force that humans inherit from their parents. We need this energy (orgasm force) to run our life each day. Each day we lose this force through sexual desire, greed, or unnecessary materialism. We need to reverse the flow of sexual energy and pump it up to the crown using the Universal Healing Tao practices of Testicle and Ovarian Breathing, Power Lock, and the Orgasmic Upward Draw. We can draw the energy through the spine to fill the three energy reservoirs: the lower tan tien (kidney and sexual centers), the middle tan tien (solar plexus and heart center), and upper tan tien (brain and Crystal Room). During its passage through the spine into the brain center, the sexual energy is transformed. After the upper reservoir is filled, the energy flows down the

palate through the tongue, and down through the throat to nourish, cool, and irrigate the heart.

2. The yin and yang waterwheel is located at the perineum (CV 1). The Boy and Girl represent the testicles and ovaries, connecting the kidneys and eyes. The Boy and Girl are working on the water treadmill, pumping the water (sexual energy) upward step by step. This movement upward, which is involved with Testicle and Ovarian Breathing, is the beginning of the Healing Love practice. By starting to roll the eyes like a ball down the front and up the back, we begin to become aware of the testicles and the ovaries rolling together with them. At the same time, we experience a loving feeling coming from the heart. Through this process the sea of sexual energy in the lower tan tien will be transformed into a lighter, more subtle force flowing upward through the spine to rejuvenate the brain, glands, and organs.

3. Pumping the water until it rises represents the yin and yang mystery (the continuous turning of the wheel by the Boy, the Girl, the testicles and the ovaries, the mind and the eyes), which will activate the great pumps (the coccyx and the sacrum) to make the water (arousal of sexual energy and orgasm) rise to "the east," the coccyx (GV 1). Even in "a lake 10,000 meters deep" (Hui Yin), the lake of sexual desire where all the yin energies of the body meet at the perineum (1), we should penetrate to the bottom; we should continue to transform these energies until our sexual desire disappears. It is from the bottom of this lake that a sweet spring flows upward to the top of the mountains after passing through the sacrum (4) (GV 2) from the perineum, up the spine to the crown, where it gushes forth like a spring fountain.

4. Sacral hiatus is the sacrum (GV 2), which has the eight immortal holes connecting directly to earth force energy.

5. The House of the Two Kidneys (GV 4) is the Ming Men or Door

of Life; it is also known as the door of fire: the gate that the sexual energy must pass through to be transformed. In Taoism we divide the left and right kidneys into yang and yin; the Ming Men is located between lumbar 2 and 3, midway between the two kidneys. The right kidney, which is yin, is represented by a Weaving Maiden who stores the essence of sexual energy (sperm and ovum), as well as the inner yang that attracts the active yang known as the Door of Life (Ming Men). The left kidney, which is yang, is known as the True Kidney, the activator of the stored energy of the kidneys. It is like a pilot light, which activates combustion in the cells of the body. It is often referred to as the Ministerial Fire, or the Genuine Fire, but is different from the Imperial Fire of the heart. We can see it as a flame bursting forth on both sides of the spine, helping to transform the energy that rises upward through its path.

6. The Burning Cauldron is located at first in the lower abdomen (below the lower tan tien, about three inches below the navel). In later practices it moves up to the heart (middle tan tien), and finally to the brain (upper tan tien). We can cook the natural forces of the mountains and rivers, the universal forces of the stars, moon, and sun, and the primordial forces of the cosmic particles, combining them within ourselves, and transforming them into a higher force to feed the Immortal Fetus.

7. The four Tai Chi symbols (yin and yang) represent the moving force (chi) of radiance. By using the mind, the eyes, and abdominal breathing, we can move the accumulated sexual energy into the cauldron and begin to cook it, transforming it into steam (chi), which will radiate throughout the channels of the entire body to repair and energize the cells. The four yin/yang symbols representing the eight trigrams of the I Ching move in balanced harmony to manifest the physical plan.

8. The Buffalo that Plows the Land and Plants the Gold Coin is located at the lower tan tien near the navel. It is connected to

the spleen, and thus to the earth. The spleen center is the seed of the spirit and the life force (chi). Once we are able to reverse the flow of sexual energy, we can irrigate the dry land, allowing us to till the soil and gather the gold to forge the gold coin of self-cultivation. Once the land is ready, the seed of long life and wisdom (the Immortal Fetus) can be planted. All the land and the plants (our soul, spirit, mind, organs, and glands) need sexual energy to grow. The stone-carving child, our pure awareness, collects the scattered parts of our essence, soul, and spirit, and strings them together into one whole.

9. The True Tan Tien, or the Field of the Elixir, is located above the Burning Cauldron in front of and below the kidneys, just behind the navel, but closer to the spine. The same area of the four Tai Chi balls is where the first alchemical transformation takes place.

10. The Weaving Maiden Spinning at her Loom is the yin (right kidney and water element), and the Cowherder standing above her at the heart level is yang. The Weaving Maiden has the ability to store silky yin energy, and to go inward to maintain quietness. She weaves silk-like garments out of moonlight and the energies of the Milky Way. These energies are accumulated and stored in the lower tan tien by using the mind, eyes, heart, and inner awareness with attention to the breathing that is gentle, soft, long, and deep. This kind of breathing, which is like spinning or pulling silk, draws in the cosmic force and weaves it into an internal chi web, or network. The Chinese legend says that the Cowherder and the Weaving Maiden were lovers once, but they neglected their duties and were changed into stars and put at opposite ends of the sky. But on the night of the seventh day of the seventh month of each year, on a day celebrated as "lover's day," the birds (magpies) make a bridge (the Milky Way) across the sky to join them together. Likewise our heart (spirit, fire, compassion fire, love, and destiny) and our

kidneys (earth nature, water, sexual energy, and physical body) have been kept separate from the day we were born. Only by reuniting the heart essence (the fire of love and compassion) and the kidney essence (sexual energy) can we give birth to and grow the Immortal Fetus.

11. Kidney spirit (Hsuan Ming), also called Nourishing the Embryo, is the ability of the kidneys to store the constitutional or inherited energy from our parents, which is fed to the inner child as it develops spiritually.

12. Within the Many Hides the Doorway to the One, located opposite the heart, which has a close relationship with the heart, and generates the big aura protecting the heart and the crown. This point is where we can draw the chi into the heart.

13. The Big Hammer, C7, is the point (big vertebra) opposite the throat. This center connects the tendons and energies from the upper and lower regions of the body. It also serves as a junction box for the nerves of the hands and legs. Any blockage at this center restricts the energy flow to the higher centers and redirects it to the hands and legs.

14. The Cave of the Spirit Peak is the Jade Pillow, located between the first cervical vertebra and the base of the skull. It is known as the "God mouth," the place where we can receive universal knowledge. This window of the sky is seen as the gateway into the Sea of Brain Marrow. This gate must open and close appropriately if energy is to pass through smoothly. The small brain, which lies within the Jade Pillow, activates yin energy that helps balance the yang energy of the large brain and serves as a storage place for the refined sexual energy and the earth force energy.

15. The Sea of Brain Marrow is connected with sexual water and spinal cord fluid; when one is drained, the other will be affected. The nine sacred mountain peaks (16 to 21) function as funnels guiding universal energy downward. This energy is then

concentrated in the mountain caves. Taoist adepts go to these caves for initiation. In the human head there are also nine different centers (peaks or points), which are able to extend to heaven to make a connection to the cosmos. The brain marrow cavity, as well as the various energy centers of the body, are like those caves in a mountain where you can concentrate, store, and transform energy.

16. Top of the Great Peak is located in the back of the head. When we tilt our head and push our chin back, our head reaches its highest point. This peak connects the North Star to the pineal gland; it is where we receive the descending universal energy (see fig. App.2).

17. The High Place of Many Veils lies between the Muddy Pool and the Great Peak. It is where the spirit and soul bodies can leave and enter into horizontal flight.

18. The Muddy Pool is located in the center of the crown (Pai Hui, or the hundredth meeting point). When it is open it feels like soft mud. This Crown point connects the Big Dipper to the hypothalamus gland. It is through this center, which functions as a two-way street, that you can project your energy (soul or spirit) upward or receive the energy flowing downward.

19. The House of Rising Yang is the third eye. Located slightly above the middle of the forehead, this center is able to receive the energies of the sun and moon, which it uses to project the soul and spirit bodies into space.

20. The Nine Sacred Realms are directly connected to the mid-eyebrow and have a close connection to the pituitary gland. This center is used to receive the cosmic force and to launch the soul and spirit bodies into the earthly or human plane for traveling.

21. The Immortal Realm is located in the center just in front of the Crown point. It is here that our energy is able to make a

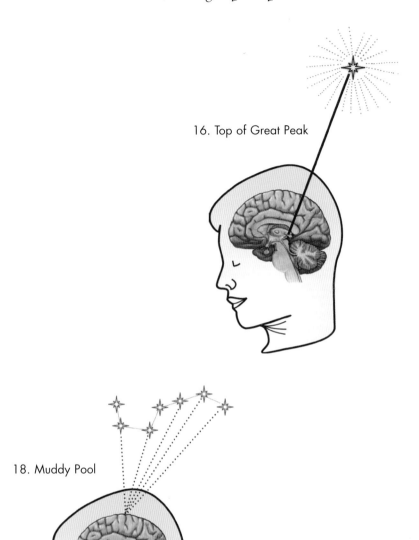

16. Top of Great Peak

18. Muddy Pool

Hypothalamus gland

Fig. App.2. Top of the Great Peak and Muddy Pool connect to the North Star and Big Dipper.

connection with the heavens to draw down even more powerful universal energies.

22. Lao Tzu (one of the founders of Taoism) is the seated figure of an old white-haired man with eyebrows reaching down to the ground, where they connect with the energy of the earth. Lao Tzu was born old, and his long eyebrows emphasize this. He embodies the one who is united with that which never dies: pure consciousness. His internal and external nature is in complete harmony and oneness with the Tao.

23. Bodhidharma (the founder of Zen Buddhism in China) is the blue-eyed standing figure holding up his hands to connect directly to the heavenly energy. The energies of Bodhidharma are mixed together with those of Lao Tzu to form a new Taoist understanding, which is the practice of modern Taoism—the Universal Healing Tao system. This system represents the blending and the harmonizing of our heavenly destiny and our earthly nature.

24. The Two Circles representing the sun and the moon within us are the left and right eyes. By learning how to roll our eyes in a circular motion, these energies, along with our sexual energy, will rise up to the crown. When we roll the eyes downward, looking toward the lower tan tien, these blended energies move down to our lower energy centers where they can be stored.

25. The Governor Channel starts at the perineum, goes up the spine to the head, then down to the palate.

26. The Conception Channel starts at the lower jaw and goes down the front of the body to the perineum.

27. The Drawbridge is the tongue, and the Pool of Water is the mouth, which holds the saliva. In the Taoist practice, when you touch the palate with the tongue (the source of rising saliva known as the Heavenly Pool), you connect the circuit between the Governor Channel (yang) and the Conception Channel

(yin). Once the tongue touches the palate, the chi is activated. The sexual energy is pumped up to the brain, activating the hypothalamus, pituitary, and thymus glands, which begin to secrete more hormones. The sexual energy, especially orgasm energy, will help draw in the heavenly force from above and the earth force from below. Mixing these two forces with the sexual energy stimulates the secretion of hormones. This creates an abundance of chi and fluid. This fluid flows like a waterfall down to the palate, then across to the back of the palate, then down to the mouth and the throat (Twelve-Storied Pagoda), where we are able to swallow it downward to fill the other two tan tiens. This water is also known as the nectar, the water of life, and the Golden Elixir.

28. The Dew Pond is located behind the soft palate and is connected to the pituitary gland. The true jade upper gate is the water gate near the throat, which connects to the brain.

29. The Mouth Pool (GV 28) is called the Mouth Crossing, which contains the elixir flowing down from the pituitary gland. This elixir can mix with the cosmic energy inhaled through the breath.

30. The Heavenly Pool (Hsuan Ying) is the source of rising saliva, which connects the tongue to the palate with the saliva.

31. The Twelve-Storied Pagoda, or Twelve-Story Tower, is the throat center (CV 22). During its passage upward through the spine into the brain center, the sexual energy is transformed. As the transformed energy continues downward from the drawbridge, it flows through the throat to nourish the heart.

32. The Flaming Balls of Fire are located at the pericardium. Cultivating our own energy field (middle tan tien or Elixir Field) means that we cultivate our own virtues—love, compassion, and kindness. Inside this field is a magical sprout (the Immortal Fetus or the unborn spirit) that "lives 10,000 years."

Its flowers—which represent the opening to consciousness and wisdom—resemble gold. These flowers never wilt. The seeds of this magical sprout are like jade pebbles. Its fruits are round. To cultivate it, we root ourselves in the earth of the Middle Palace (the solar plexus). To water it, we reverse the sexual energy so it flows upward to the crown. The text says: "After many years, I achieve the Great Tao and wander freely over the earth; I am an Immortal of the story Island of Peng Lai (the High Astral Plane)."

33. The Spiral of Rice Grains represents the great mystery: the world in a grain of sand, the microcosm of the human organism reflecting the macrocosm of the universe. Once we learn to understand and control our mind and ourselves, we will understand the mysteries and laws of the universe. The Law of Heaven is called destiny, and the Law of Earth is called nature. The harmony between destiny and nature is the Tao, the Great Way. Those who follow the Tao fulfill their spiritual destiny and enjoy the fruit of their earthly nature. The Taoist way of life is to tap into the energies of Heaven and Earth while blending and harmonizing these energies with the human energy in order to cultivate and conserve the vital force in our bodies. Heavenly forces manifest themselves as celestial energy whose power appears to us as thoughts, consciousness, fate, and destiny. Some systems and religions separate Heaven and Earth, making us choose between them, while the Universal Healing Tao is the practice of connecting and harmonizing Heaven (destiny) and Earth (nature) in our own being.

34. The Cowherder Boy connecting the stars symbolizes the yang elements of the heart: the fire of love and the fire of compassion. The Cowherder looks like a child, which we call yang heart or Heart spirit (Tan Yuan). He is also called Guarding Spirit. Both the Christian Bible and ancient Taoist texts refer to this transformation as "becoming like a child again": the symbol of

spiritual wisdom, innocence, and simplicity. Extending out of the Cowherder's crown is the Big Dipper, which symbolizes the heart's quest to seek harmony with the cosmos. Taoists regard the Big Dipper as the cosmic timepiece. During the course of the year, the Big Dipper makes a 360-degree rotation, pointing to all the stars, collecting the universal power in the Big Dipper's cup. If we know how to make the connection with the Big Dipper we can easily gather the astral power for our own transformation.

35. The Milky Way (or Magpie Bridge) is the bridge made of birds (magpies) connecting the Cowherder (the heart, the fire of love) to the Weaving Maiden (the kidneys, the water of sexual energy).

36. The Lung spirit (Hwa Hao) finds "fullness in the empty is completed": the power and ability of the lungs to empty themselves so they can receive more. Each inhalation and exhalation of our body is the breath of the universe expanding and contracting.

37. The Middle Palace, the solar plexus, is also known as the middle tan tien.

38. The Outer Ring of the Forest represents the edge of the rib cage, where the diaphragm is anchored.

39. The Liver spirit (Lung Yien), also called Growing Wisdom, is the connection of the forest of trees to the liver (wood element), the largest organ of the body. In Taoism, we regard the liver as the controller of the chi and blood. Too much chi in one place can cause stagnation or congestion, and too little can cause weakness and depletion. Both conditions are the result of a liver imbalance. The Weaving Maiden (kidneys), who receives water from the sexual energy, also makes water, which helps the wood (liver) to grow while the liver provides fuel for the heart's fire. The organs all depend on one another.

39a. The Gall Bladder spirit (Lung Au), also called Majestic and Bright, is located in the middle of the liver.

39b. The Spleen spirit (Chaeng Tsai), also called Soul Pavilion, is located in the spleen area.

40. Includes a Boy Plowing with a Buffalo, the Burning Cauldron (6), and the moving of the four yin and yang (Tai Chi) balls (7).

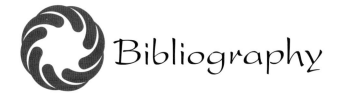

Bibliography

Aihara, Herman. *Acid and Alkaline*. Chico, Calif.: Oshawa Macrobiotic Foundation, 1986.

Aivanhov, Omraam. *Spiritual Alchemy*. Newburyport, Mass.: Red Wheel Weiser Books, 1989.

Alder, Vera Stanley. *The Finding of the Third Eye*. Newburyport, Mass.: Weiser Books, 1980.

Alexanderson, Olga. *Living Water*. New York: Gill and Company, 2002.

Allen, James. *As a Man Thinketh*. New York: TarcherPerigee/Penguin, 2006.

Andersen, Jefferson. *Sun Sign Moon Sign*. Los Angeles: International Books, 1967.

Bach, Richard. *Jonathan Livingston Seagull*. New York: Scribner, 2006.

Bakhru, H. K. *Food that Heals*. New Delhi: Orient Paperbacks, 1995.

Barker, Sarah. *The Alexander Technique*. New York: Bantam, 1979.

Barnard, Neal D. *The Power of Your Plate*. Summertown, Tenn.: Book Publishing Company, 1990.

Bastiat, Frederic. *The Law*. New York: Martino Fine Books, 2011.

Bates, William. *Better Eyesight without Glasses*. New York: Holt Paperbacks, 1981.

Bealle, Morris Allison. *The Drug Story*. Whitefish, Mont.: Literary Licensing LLC, 1949.

Beattie, Melody. *Codependence No More*. Center City, Minn.: Hazelden, 1986.

Becker, Robert, and Gary Selden. *The Body Electric*. New York: William Morrow Paperbacks, 1998.

Beecher, Willard. *Beyond Success and Failure*. Camarillo, Calif.: DeVorss and Company, 1986.

Blofeld, John. *The Secret and Sublime: Taoist Mysteries and Magic*. New York: Dutton, 1973.

———. *Taoism: Road to Immortality*. Boston: Shambhala, 2000.

Bly, Robert. *Iron John*. New York: Da Capo Press, 2004.

Boone, J. Allen. *The Language of Silence*. New York: Joanna Cotler Books, 1976.

Bradshaw, John. *Healing the Shame that Binds You,* rev. ed. Deerfield Beach, Florida: HCI, 2005.

Bragg, Paul. *Apple Cider Vinegar*. Santa Barbara, Calif.: Bragg Health Sciences, 2005.

Brann, W. C. *The Iconoclast*. New York: Forgotten Books, 2015.

Burkins, Lee. *Soldier's Heart*. Bloomington, Ind.: Author's House, 2003.

Camp, Robert Lee. *Love Cards*. Concord, Calif.: Seven Thunders Publishing, 2004.

Campbell, Joseph. *Myths to Live By*. New York: Penguin Books, 1993.

Capra, Fritjof. *The Tao of Physics*. Boston: Shambhala, 2010.

———. *The Web of Life*. New York: Anchor, 1997.

Carson, Rachel. *Silent Spring*. New York: Houghton Mifflin Company, 2002.

Carson, Robert. *Taming Your Gremlin*. New York: William Morrow Paperbacks, 2003.

Carter, Al. *Rebound Exercise*. Calif.: Rebound Intl., 1979.

Castaneda, Carlos. *Journey to Ixtlan*. New York: Washington Square Press, 1991.

———. *Tales of Power*. New York: Washington Square Press, 1991.

Cayce, Edgar. *Astrology and Cayce*. Virginia Beach, Va.: A.R.E. Foundation, 1946.

———. *The Book of Revelation: A Commentary Based on a Study of Twenty-Three Psychic Discourses by Edgar Cayce*. Virginia Beach, Va.: A.R.E. Press, 1995.

Chang, Stephen Thomas. *The Tao of Sexology*. San Francisco: Tao Publishing, 1986.

———. *The Great Tao*. San Francisco: Tao Publishing, 1985.

Chia, Mantak. *Advanced Chi Nei Tsang: Enhancing Chi Energy in the Vital Organs*. Rochester, Vt.: Destiny Books, 2009.

———. *The Alchemy of Sexual Energy: Connecting to the Universe from Within*. Rochester, Vt.: Destiny Books, 2009.

———. *Bone Marrow Nei Kung: Taoist Techniques for Rejuvenating the Blood and Bone*. Rochester, Vt.: Destiny Books, 2006.

———. *Chi Nei Tsang: Chi Massage for the Vital Organs*. Rochester, Vt.: Destiny Books, 2007.

———. *Chi Self-Massage: The Taoist Way of Rejuvenation*. Rochester, Vt.: Destiny Books, 2006.

———. *Cosmic Fusion: The Inner Alchemy of the Eight Forces*. Rochester, Vt.: Destiny Books, 2007.

———. *Energy Balance through the Tao: Exercises for Cultivating Yin Energy*. Rochester, Vt.: Destiny Books, 2005.

———. *Fusion of the Eight Psychic Channels: Opening and Sealing the Energy Body*. Rochester, Vt.: Destiny Books, 2008.

———. *Fusion of the Five Elements: Meditations for Transforming Negative Emotions*. Rochester, Vt.: Destiny Books, 2007.

———. *Golden Elixir Chi Kung*. Rochester, Vt.: Destiny Books, 2005.

———. *The Healing Energy of Shared Consciousness: A Taoist Approach to Entering the Universal Mind*. Rochester, Vt.: Destiny Books, 2011.

———. *Healing Light of the Tao: Foundational Practices to Awaken Chi Energy*. Rochester, Vt.: Destiny Books, 2008.

———. *Healing Love through the Tao: Cultivating Female Sexual Energy*. Rochester, Vt.: Destiny Books, 2005.

———. *The Inner Smile: Increasing Chi through the Cultivation of Joy*. Rochester, Vt.: Destiny Books, 2008.

———. *Iron Shirt Chi Kung*. Rochester, Vt.: Destiny Books, 2006.

———. *Karsai Nei Tsang: Therapeutic Massage for the Sexual Organs*. Rochester, Vt.: Destiny Books, 2011.

———. *The Six Healing Sounds: Taoist Techniques for Balancing Chi*. Rochester, Vt.: Destiny Books, 2009.

———. *Tan Tien Chi Kung: Foundational Exercises for Empty Force and Perineum Power*. Rochester, Vt.: Destiny Books, 2004.

———. *Taoist Cosmic Healing: Chi Kung Color Healing Principles for*

Detoxification and Rejuvenation. Rochester, Vt.: Destiny Books, 2003.

———. *The Taoist Soul Body: Harnessing the Power of Kan and Li.* Rochester, Vt.: Destiny Books, 2007.

———. *Tendon Nei Kung: Building Strength, Power, and Flexibility in the Joints.* Rochester, Vt.: Destiny Books, 2009.

———. *Wisdom Chi Kung: Practices for Enlivening the Brain with Chi Energy.* Rochester, Vt.: Destiny Books, 2008.

Chia, Mantak, and Douglas Abrams. *The Multi-Orgasmic Man: Sexual Secrets Every Man Should Know.* New York: HarperCollins, 1996.

———. *The Multi-Orgasmic Couple: Sexual Secrets Every Couple Should Know.* New York: HarperCollins, 2000.

Chia, Mantak, and Rachel Carlton Abrams. *The Multi-Orgasmic Woman: Sexual Secrets Every Woman Should Know.* New York: HarperCollins, 2005.

———. Chia, Mantak, and Christine Harkness-Giles. *Inner Alchemy Astrology: Practical Techniques for Controlling Your Destiny.* Rochester, Vt.: Destiny Books, 2013.

———. *Pi Gu Chi Kung: Inner Alchemy Energy Fasting.* Rochester, Vt.: Destiny Books, 2016.

Chia, Mantak, and Lee Holden. *Simple Chi Kung: Exercises for Awakening the Life-Force Energy.* Rochester, Vt.: Destiny Books, 2011.

Chia, Mantak, and Tao Huang. *The Secret Teachings of the Tao Te Ching.* Rochester, Vt.: Destiny Books, 2005.

Chia, Mantak, and Andrew Jan. *Greatest Kan and Li: Gathering the Cosmic Light.* Rochester, Vt.: Destiny Books, 2014.

———. *The Practice of Greater Kan and Li: Techniques for Creating the Immortal Self.* Rochester, Vt.: Destiny Books, 2014.

———. *Tai Chi Fa Jin: Advanced Techniques for Discharging Chi Energy.* Rochester, Vt.: Destiny Books, 2012.

———. *Tai Chi Wu Style: Advanced Techniques for Internalizing Chi Energy.* Rochester, Vt.: Destiny Books, 2013.

Chia, Mantak, and Robert T. Lewanski. *The Art of Cosmic Vision: Practices for Improving Your Eyesight.* Rochester, Vt.: Destiny Books, 2010.

Chia, Mantak, and Juan Li. *The Inner Structure of Tai Chi: Mastering the Classic Forms of Tai Chi Chi Kung.* Rochester, Vt.: Destiny Books, 2005.

Chia, Mantak, and Kris Deva North. *Taoist Foreplay: Love Meridians and Pressure Points*. Rochester, Vt.: Destiny Books, 2010.

———. *Taoist Shaman: Practices from the Wheel of Life*. Rochester, Vt.: Destiny Books, 2011.

Chia, Mantak, and Dirk Oellibrandt. *Taoist Astral Healing: Chi Kung Healing Practices Using Star and Planet Energies*. Rochester, Vt.: Destiny Books, 2004.

Chia, Mantak, and Dena Saxer. *Emotional Wisdom: Daily Tools for Transforming Anger, Depression, and Fear*. Novato, Calif.: New World Library, 2009.

Chia, Mantak, and Aisha Sieburth. *Life Pulse Massage: Taoist Techniques for Enhanced Circulation and Detoxification*. Rochester, Vt.: Destiny Books, 2015.

Chia, Mantak, and Joyce Thom. *Craniosacral Chi Kung: Integrating Body and Emotion in the Cosmic Flow*. Rochester, Vt.: Destiny Books, 2016.

Chia, Mantak, and William U. Wei. *Basic Practices of the Universal Healing Tao: An Illustrated Guide to Levels 1 through 6*. Rochester, Vt.: Destiny Books, 2013.

———. *Chi Kung for Prostate Health and Sexual Vigor: A Handbook of Simple Exercises and Techniques*. Rochester, Vt.: Destiny Books, 2013.

———. *Chi Kung for Women's Health and Sexual Vitality: A Handbook of Simple Exercises and Techniques*. Rochester, Vt.: Destiny Books, 2014.

———. *Chi Nei Ching: Muscle, Tendon, and Meridian Massage*. Rochester, Vt.: Destiny Books, 2013.

———. *Cosmic Astrology: An East-West Guide to Your Energy Persona*. Rochester, Vt.: Destiny Books, 2012.

———. *Cosmic Detox: A Taoist Approach to Internal Cleansing*. Rochester, Vt.: Destiny Books, 2011.

———. *Cosmic Nutrition: The Taoist Approach to Health and Longevity*. Rochester, Vt.: Destiny Books, 2012.

———. *Living in the Tao: The Effortless Path of Self-Discovery*. Rochester, Vt.: Destiny Books, 2009.

———. *Sealing of the Five Senses: Advanced Practices for Becoming a Taoist Immortal*. Rochester, Vt.: Destiny Books, 2014.

————. *Sexual Reflexology: Activating the Taoist Points of Love.* Rochester, Vt.: Destiny Books, 2003.

Chia, Mantak, and Michael Winn. *Taoist Secrets of Love: Cultivating Male Sexual Energy.* Santa Fe, N.M.: Aurora Press, 1984.

Chopra, Deepak. *Quantum Healing.* New York: Bantam, 1990.

————. *Way of the Wizard.* New York: Harmony, 1995.

Clark, Hulda. *Cure for all Diseases.* Chula Vista, Calif.: New Century Press, 1995.

Cleary, Thomas. *I Ching.* Boston: Shambhala, 2006.

————. *Inner Teachings of Taoism.* Boston: Shambhala, 2001.

————. *Opening the Dragon's Gate.* North Clarendon, Vt.: Tuttle Publishing, 1998.

————. *Spirit of Tao.* Boston: Shambhala, 1993.

————. *Taoist I Ching.* Boston: Shambhala, 2005.

Chung, T. C. *Sayings of Lieh Tzu.* Ariz.: El Paso Norte Press, 2011.

Cohen, Kenneth S. *The Way of Qigong.* New York.: Wellspring/Ballantine, 1999.

Cousens, Gabriel. *Spiritual Nutrition and the Rainbow Diet.* Boulder, Colo.: Cassandra Press, 1986.

Danaos, Kosta. *The Magus of Java.* Rochester, Vt.: Inner Traditions, 2000.

Deida, David. *Way of the Superior Man.* Louisville, Colo.: Sounds True, 2004.

Douglas, Nik, and Penny Slinger. *Sexual Secrets.* Rochester, Vt.: Destiny Books, 1999.

Eckermann, Johann. *Words of Goethe.* New York: Tudor, 1949.

Ehret, Arnold. *Arnold Ehret's Mucusless Diet Healing System.* New York: Benedict Lust Publications, 2015.

Evatt, Cris, and Bruce Feld. *The Givers and the Takers.* Sausalito, Calif.: Papaya Press, 2008.

Farrell, Warren. *The Liberated Man.* New York: Berkley/Penguin, 1993.

Fleming, Candace. *Ben Franklin's Almanac: Being a True Account of the Good Gentleman's Life.* New York: Atheneum Books for Young Readers, 2003.

Franklin, Ben. *Poor Richard's Almanac,* repr. ed. White Plains, New York: Peter Pauper Press, 1981.

Frantzis, Bruce. *The Great Stillness*. Berkeley, Calif.: North Atlantic Books, 2001.

Friedman, Milton. *Free to Choose*. New York: Mariner Books, 1990.

Geller, Uri. *Mind Medicine*. Rockport, Mass.: Element Books, 1999.

Goldberg, Herb. *The Hazards of Being Male*. New York: Signet, 1977.

Golding, William. *Lord of the Flies*. New York: Penguin Books, 2003.

Graham, A. C. *The Book of Lieh-Tzu*. New York: Columbia University Press, 1990.

Gray, Henry. *Gray's Anatomy*. New York: Gramercy Books, 1988.

Gray, John. *Men Are from Mars and Women Are from Venus*. New York: Harper Paperbacks, 2012.

Gregory, Dick. *Dick Gregory's Natural Diet for Folks Who Eat*. New York: Harper and Row Publishers, 1974.

Hall, Manley P. *America's Assignment with Destiny*. Los Angeles: Philosophical Research Society, 1994.

———. *The Secret Teachings of All Ages*. New York: TarcherPerigee/Penguin, 2003.

Heinlein, Robert. *Stranger in a Strange Land*. New York: Ace Books, 1991.

Hesse, Hermann. *Siddhartha*. New York: Bantam Books, 1981.

———. *Steppenwolf*. New York: Penguin Books, 1999.

Hicks, Karen. *The Tao of an Uncluttered Life*. Lake Worth, Fl.: Green Dragon Publishing Group, 1999.

Hill, Napoleon. *Think and Grow Rich*. New York: Create Space Independent Publishing Platform, 2010.

Hill, Napoleon, and Clement Stone. *Success through a Positive Mental Attitude*. New York: Pocket Books, 1977.

Hinn, Benny. *The Anointing*. Nashville, Tenn.: Thomas Nelson, 1997.

Hoff, Benjamin. *The Tao of Pooh*. New York: Penguin Books, 1983.

Jarves, D. C. *Folk Medicine*. New York: Holt, Rhinehart and Winston, 1958.

Jasmuheen. *Living on Light*. Frankfurt am Main, Germany: KOHA Publishing, 1998.

Jensen, Bernard. *The Chemistry of Man*. Warsaw, Ind.: Whitman Publications, 2007.

———. *The Healing Power of Chlorophyll from Plant Life*. Escondido, Calif.: Jensen Enterprises, 1973.

————. *The Science and Practice of Iridology*. Warsaw, Ind.: Whitman Publications, 2005.

Jensen, Bernard, and Mark Anderson. *Empty Harvest,* repr. ed. New York: Avery, 1995.

Jung, Carl. *Memories, Dreams, Reflections*. New York: Vintage, 1989.

Kelder, Peter. *Ancient Secret of the Fountain of Youth*. New York: Doubleday Religion, 1998.

Keys, Ken. *The Hundredth Monkey*. Camarillo, Calif.: Devorss and Co., 1984.

Kim, Joseph K. *Compass of Health*. Encino, Calif.: Heal and Soul, 2010.

King, Stephen. *On Writing*. New York: Pocket Books, 2002.

Kit, Wong Kiew. *The Art of Chi Kung*. Los Angeles: Cosmos Internet, 2014.

Klaper, Michael. *Vegan Nutrition,* 4th ed. Kapaau, Hawaii: Gentle World, 1997.

Koestler, Arthur. *The Thirteenth Tribe*. New York: Popular Library, 1978.

Koh, Vincent. *Hsia Calendar: 1924–2024*. Singapore: Asiapac Books, 1998.

Kohn, Livia. *The Taoist Experience*. Albany: State University of New York Press, 1993.

Kostrubala, Thaddeus. *The Joy of Running*. Calif.: Saint Nicholas Productions, 2013.

Krishnamurti, Jiddu. *Commentaries on Living*. Wheaton, Ill.: Quest Books. 1956.

Kroeger, Hanna. *Ageless Remedies from Mother's Kitchen*. Boulder, Colo.: Hanna Kroeger Publications, 1981.

————. *Arteriosclerosis and Herbal Chelation*. Boulder, Colo.: Hanna Kroeger Publications, 1984.

————. *Old Time Remedies*. Boulder, Colo.: Hanna Kroeger Publications, 2006.

————. *Parasites: The Enemy Within*. Boulder, Colo.: Hanna Kroeger Publications, 2005.

Krystal, Jim. *Taming our Monkey Mind*. New York: Weiser Books, 1994.

Kushi, Michio. *Book of Do-In*. Tokyo: Japan Publications, 1979.

————. *Natural Healing*. Japan: Kodansha, 1979.

————. *Spiral of Life*. Becket, Mass.: East West Foundation, 1978.

Lad, Vasant D. *Secrets of the Pulse,* 2nd. ed. Albuquerque: Ayurvedic Press, 2006.

LaLanne, Jack. *The Jack LaLanne Way to Vibrant Good Health.* Upper Saddle River, N.J.: Prentice Hall, 1961.

Lash, John. *The Tai Chi Journey.* Rockport, Mass.: Element Books, 1997.

Lawlor, Robert. *Sacred Geometry.* London: Thames and Hudson, 1982.

Lu, Henry C. *Chinese Foods for Longevity.* New York: Sterling Publishing Co., 1990.

Mahesh, Maharishi. *Maharishi Mahesh Yogi on the Bhagavad Gita,* repr. ed. New York: Penguin Books, 1990.

Mandino, Og. *Greatest Salesman in the World.* New York: Bantam, 1969.

Man Ho, Kwok, and Joanne O'Brien. *The Eight Immortals of Taoism.* New York: Plume, 1991.

Mann, John, and Lar Short. *The Body of Light.* North Clarendon, Vt.: Tuttle Publishing, 1993.

Markides, Kyriacos. *The Magus of Stovolos.* New York: Penguin Books, 1989.

Melchizedeck, Drunvalo. *The Ancient Secret of the Flower of Life.* Flagstaff, Ariz.: Light Technology Publishing, 2000.

Mendelsohn, Robert S. *Confessions of a Medical Heretic.* Chicago: Contemporary Books; 1979.

———. *Male Practice: How Doctors Manipulate Women,* rev. ed. Chicago: Contemporary Books, 1982.

Merton, Thomas. *The Way of Chuang Tzu,* 2nd. ed. New York: New Directions, 2010.

Millman, Dan. *Way of the Peaceful Warrior.* Novato, Calif.: HJ Kramer, 2006.

Milne, A. A. *Pooh's Pot o' Honey.* New York: Dutton, 1968.

Ming-Dao, Deng. *Chronicles of Tao.* New York: Harper One, 1993.

———. *The Wandering Taoist.* New York: Harper and Row, 1986.

Ming, Lui. *Awakening to the Tao.* Translated by Thomas Cleary. Boston: Shambhala, 2006.

Misita, Michael. *Believing in Nothing.* Malibu, Calif.: Valley of the Sun Publishing Co., 1994

Missildine, Marilyn. *Your Inner Child of the Past*. New York: Pocket Books, 1991.

Montessori, Maria. *The Secret of Childhood*. New York: Ballantine Books, 1982.

Mullins, Eustace. *Murder by Injection*. Omnia Veritas, 2016.

Murphy, Joseph. *Secrets of the I Ching*. New York: Prentice Hall, 1999.

Nietzsche, Frederic. *The Anti-Christ*. New York: SoHo Books, 2013.

Ni, Hua-Ching. *Complete Works of Lao Tzu*. Ashland, Ohio: Seven Star Communications, 1995.

———. *Eight Thousand Years of Wisdom*. Ashland, Ohio: Seven Star Communications, 1985.

O'Malley, William. *The Fifth Week,* 2nd ed. Chicago: Loyola Press, 1998.

Orr, Leonard. *Breaking the Death Habit*. New York: Frog Books, 1998.

———. *Physical Immortality*. New York: Inspiration University, 1988.

Osho. *The Book of Nothing: Han Hsin Ming*. New York: Osho, 2009.

———. *Tao of the Pathless Path*. Canada: Renaissance Books, 2002.

Ouspensky, P. D. *The Fourth Way*. New York: Vintage, 1971.

Page, Michael. *The Tao of Power*. Fairview, N.C.: Green Print, 1989.

Palmer, Martin. *The Book of Chuang Tzu*. New York: Penguin Classics, 2007.

———. *The Elements of Taoism*. Rockport, Mass.: Element Books, 1997.

Paracelsus. *Alchemical Catechism*. Sequim, Wash.: Holmes Publishing Group, 1983.

Peale, Norman Vincent. *The Power of Positive Thinking*. Palmer, Alaska: Fireside Books, 2007.

Peck, Scott. *The Road Less Traveled*. New York: Simon and Schuster, 1978.

Peck, Stephen. *Atlas of Human Anatomy*. New York: Oxford University Press, 1982.

Powell, John. *Why Am I Afraid to Love?* Merrimack, N.H.: Thomas More Press, 1995.

Rajneesh, Bhagwan Shree. *The Book of Secrets*. New York: St. Martin's Press, 1982.

———. *Tao: The Three Treasures,* vol. 1. New York: Rajneesh Foundation Intl., 1983.

Rampa, T. Lobsang. *Chapters of Life*. New York: Corgi Books, 1977.

Ramtha. *I Am Ramtha,* 3rd ed. Hillsboro, Ore.: Beyond Words Publishing Co., 1986.

Robbins, John. *Diet for a New America.* Novato, Calif.: HJ Kramer, 1998.

Roberts, Henry C. *The Complete Prophecies of Nostradamus.* New York: Three Rivers Press, 1994.

Roberts, Monty. *The Man Who Listens to Horses.* New York: Ballantine Books, 2008.

Ruffin, C. Bernard. *Padre Pio: The True Story.* Huntington, Ind.: Our Sunday Visitor, 1982.

Sacks, Robert. *Nine Star Ki.* Bloomington, Ind.: iUniverse, 2008.

Saraydarian, Torkom. *Irritation: The Destructive Fire.* Cave Creek, Ariz.: T.S.G. Publishing Foundation, 1992.

———. *The Science of Meditation.* Cave Creek, Ariz.: TSG Publishing Foundation, 1976.

Schaef, Arthur. *When Society Becomes an Addict.* New York: Harper One, 1988.

Schlessinger, John. *Things Women Do.* New York: Harper Perennial, 2002.

Schopenhauer, Arthur. *Essays and Aphorisms.* New York: Penguin Classic, 1973.

Schwarz, Jack. *Human Energy Systems.* New York: Penguin Books, 1992.

———. *It's Not What You Eat but What Eats You.* Berkeley, Calif.: Celestial Arts, 1995.

———. *The Path of Action.* New York: Plume, 1977.

———. *Voluntary Controls.* New York: Plume, 1978.

Shelton, Herbert M. *The Science and Fine Arts of Fasting.* Eastford, Ct.: Martino Fine Books Publishing, 2013.

———. *Health for the Millions,* 2nd ed. Youngstown, Ohio: National Health Assoc., 1996.

Shih, T. K. *The Swimming Dragon.* New York: Station Hill Press, 1999.

Singer, Blair. *Sales Dogs.* Cleveland, Ohio: RDA Press, 2012.

Sitchin, Zecharia. *The Twelfth Planet.* Rochester, Vt.: Bear & Company, 1991.

———. *Stairway to Heaven.* Rochester, Vt.: Bear & Company, 1992.

Smullyan, Raymond. *The Tao Is Silent.* New York: Harper One; Reissue edition, 1977.

Spalding, Warren. *Life and Teachings of the Masters of the Far East,* 6 vols., rev. ed. Camarillo, Calif.: Devorss and Co., 1986.

Stone, Diane. *The Tao of Inner Peace.* New York: Plume, 2000.

Sun Bear. *Buffalo Hearts.* Happy Camp, Calif.: Naturegraph Publishers, 1970.

Thoreau, Henry David. *Reflections at Walden: Selected Writings of Henry David Thoreau with Color Photographs Taken at Walden Pond.* Edited by Peter Seymour and James Morgan. Kansas City, Mo.: Hallmark, 1971.

———. *Walden.* Princeton: Princeton University Press, 2004.

Tilden, John H. *Toxemia Explained.* Minneapolis: Filiquarian Publishing, 2007.

Tolken, J. R. R. *The Hobbit.* New York: Houghton Mifflin, 2002.

Tolle, Eckhart. *The Power of Now.* Vancouver, Canada: Namaste Publishing, 2004.

———. *Stillness Speaks.* London: Hodder and Stoughton, 2003.

Tompkins, Peter, and Christopher Bird. *The Secret Life of Plants.* New York: Harper Perennial, 1989.

———. *Secrets of the Soil.* Eagle River, Alaska: Earthpulse Press, 1998.

Tortora, Gerard J., and Grabowski, Sandra Reynolds. *Introduction to the Human Body.* New York: John Wiley and Sons, 2001.

———. *Principles of Anatomy and Physiology.* New York: McGraw-Hill, 1999.

Towler, Solala. *Embracing the Way: A Guide to Western Taoism.* Eugene, Ore.: Abode of the Eternal Tao, 1998.

Tsatsouline, Pavel. *Beyond Stretching,* 2nd ed. Little Canada, Minn.: Dragon Door Publications, 1998.

Tzu, Sun. *Art of War.* Boston: Shambhala, 2005.

Wallach, Joel D., and Ma Lan. *Rare Earths Forbidden Cures.* Body Basics, 2000.

Wapnick, Kenneth. *Forgiveness and Jesus,* 6th ed. Temecula, Calif.: Foundation for "A Course in Miracles," 1998.

Watts, Allen. *Beyond Theology: The Art of Godmanship.* New York: Vintage, 1973.

———. *The Book: On the Taboo Against Knowing Who You Are.* New York: Vintage, 1989.

———. *Nature, Man and Woman.* New York: Vintage, 1991.

Webster, Dennis. *Acidophilus and Colon Health.* Denver: NutriBooks, 1984.

Wei, Wu. *I Ching Wisdom.* Malibu, Calif.: Power Press, 2005.

Wigmore, Ann. *The Wheat Grass Book.* New York: Avery Publishing Group, 1984.

Whiteside, Robert. *Agile at 80.* Hawaii: Self-Published, 1989.

Wong, Eva. *Cultivating Stillness.* Boston: Shambhala, 1992.

———. *Harmonizing Yin and Yang.* Boston: Shambhala, 1997.

———. *Tales of the Taoist Immortals.* Boston: Shambhala, 2001.

———. *The Tao of Health, Longevity, and Immortality: The Teachings of Immortals Chung and Lü.* Boston: Shambhala, 2000.

———. *Taoism: An Essential Guide.* Boston: Shambhala, 2011.

Yogananda, Paramahansa. *Autobiography of a Yogi.* Los Angeles: Self-Realization Fellowship Publishers, 1994.

Young, Robert O., and Shelley Redford Young. *Sick and Tired? Reclaim Your Inner Terrain.* Salt Lake City: Woodland Publishing, 2001.

Yu, Anthony. *Journey to the West,* 4 vols. China: Foreign Languages Press, 2003.

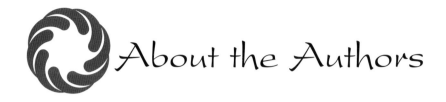

About the Authors

MANTAK CHIA

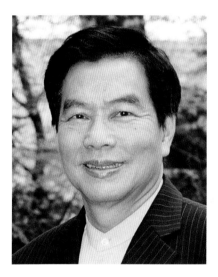

Mantak Chia has been studying the Taoist approach to life since childhood. His mastery of this ancient knowledge, enhanced by his study of other disciplines, has resulted in the development of the Universal Healing Tao system, which is now being taught throughout the world.

Mantak Chia was born in Thailand to Chinese parents in 1944. When he was six years old, he learned from Buddhist monks how to sit and "still the mind." While in grammar school he learned traditional Thai boxing, and he soon went on to acquire considerable skill in aikido, yoga, and Tai Chi. His studies of the Taoist way of life began in earnest when he was a student in Hong Kong, ultimately leading to his mastery of a wide variety of esoteric disciplines, with the guidance of several masters, including Master I Yun, Master Meugi, Master Cheng Yao Lun, and Master Pan Yu. To better understand the mechanisms behind healing energy, he also studied Western anatomy and medical sciences.

Master Chia has taught his system of healing and energizing practices to tens of thousands of students and trained more than two thousand instructors and practitioners throughout the world. He has established centers for Taoist study and training in many countries around the globe. In June of 1990, he was honored by the International Congress of Chinese Medicine and Qi Gong (Chi Kung), which named him the Qi Gong Master of the Year.

WILLIAM U. WEI

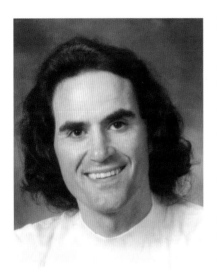

Born after World War II, growing up in the Midwest area of the United States, and trained in Catholicism, William Wei became a student of the Tao and started studying under Master Mantak Chia in the early 1980s. In the later 1980s he became a senior instructor of the Universal Healing Tao, specializing in one-on-one training. In the early 1990s William Wei moved to Tao Garden, Thailand, and assisted Master Mantak Chia in building Tao Garden Taoist Training Center. For six years William traveled to over thirty countries, teaching with Master Mantak Chia and serving as marketing and construction coordinator for the Tao Garden. Upon completion of Tao Garden in December 2000, he became project manager for all the Universal Tao publications and products. With the purchase of a mountain with four waterfalls in southern Oregon, USA, in the late 1990s, William Wei is presently completing a Taoist Mountain Sanctuary for personal cultivation, higher-level practices, and ascension (see his website: **www.wuchifoundation.org**). William Wei is the coauthor with Master Chia of *Sexual Reflexology, Living in the Tao, Basic Practices of the Universal Healing Tao, Chi Nei Ching,* and the

Taoist poetry book of 366 daily poems, *Emerald River,* which expresses the feeling, essence, and stillness of the Tao. The Professor—Master of Nothingness, the Myth that takes the Mystery out of Mysticism, William U. Wei, also known as Wei Tzu, is a pen name for this instructor so the instructor can remain anonymous and can continue to become a blade of grass in a field of grass.

The Universal Healing Tao System and Training Center

THE UNIVERSAL HEALING TAO SYSTEM

The ultimate goal of Taoist practice is to transcend physical boundaries through the development of the soul and the spirit within the human. That is also the guiding principle behind the Universal Healing Tao, a practical system of self-development that enables individuals to complete the harmonious evolution of their physical, mental, and spiritual bodies. Through a series of ancient Chinese meditative and internal energy exercises, the practitioner learns to increase physical energy, release tension, improve health, practice self-defense, and gain the ability to heal him- or herself and others. In the process of creating a solid foundation of health and well-being in the physical body, the practitioner also creates the basis for developing his or her spiritual potential by learning to tap into the natural energies of the sun, moon, earth, stars, and other environmental forces.

The Universal Healing Tao practices are derived from ancient techniques rooted in the processes of nature. They have been gathered and integrated into a coherent, accessible system for well-being that works directly with the life force, or chi, that flows through the meridian system of the body.

Master Chia has spent years developing and perfecting techniques for teaching these traditional practices to students around the world through ongoing classes, workshops, private instruction, and healing sessions, as well as books and video and audio products. Further information can be obtained at www.universal-tao.com.

THE UNIVERSAL HEALING TAO TRAINING CENTER

The Tao Garden Resort and Training Center in northern Thailand is the home of Master Chia and serves as the worldwide headquarters for Universal Healing Tao activities. This integrated wellness, holistic health, and training center is situated on eighty acres surrounded by the beautiful Himalayan foothills near the historic walled city of Chiang Mai. The serene setting includes flower and herb gardens ideal for meditation, open-air pavilions for practicing Chi Kung, and a health and fitness spa.

The center offers classes year round, as well as summer and winter retreats. It can accommodate two hundred students, and group leasing can be arranged. For information on courses, books, products, and other resources, see below.

RESOURCES

Universal Healing Tao Center
274 Moo 7, Luang Nua, Doi Saket, Chiang Mai, 50220 Thailand
Tel: (66)(53) 921-200
Email: universaltao@universal-tao.com
Website: www.universal-tao.com

For information on retreats and the health spa, contact:
Tao Garden Health Spa & Resort
Email: reservations@tao-garden.com
Website: www.tao-garden.com

Good Chi • Good Heart • Good Intention

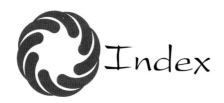# Index

BOOKS OF RELATED INTEREST

The Eight Immortal Healers
Taoist Wisdom for Radiant Health
by Mantak Chia and Johnathon Dao, M.D. (A.M.), L.Ac.

EMDR and the Universal Healing Tao
An Energy Psychology Approach to
Overcoming Emotional Trauma
by Mantak Chia and Doug Hilton

Healing Love through the Tao
Cultivating Female Sexual Energy
by Mantak Chia

Chi Self-Massage
The Taoist Way of Rejuvenation
by Mantak Chia

Craniosacral Chi Kung
Integrating Body and Emotion in the Cosmic Flow
by Mantak Chia and Joyce Thom

Chi Kung for Prostate Health and Sexual Vigor
A Handbook of Simple Exercises and Techniques
by Mantak Chia and William U. Wei

Healing Light of the Tao
Foundational Practices to Awaken Chi Energy
by Mantak Chia

Iron Shirt Chi Kung
by Mantak Chia

INNER TRADITIONS • BEAR & COMPANY
P.O. Box 388 • Rochester, VT 05767
1-800-246-8648
www.InnerTraditions.com

Or contact your local bookseller